100 Questions & Answers About Melanoma and Other Skin Cancers

Edward F. McClay, MD
Mary-Eileen T. McClay
Jodie Smith

JONES AND BARTLETT PUBLISHERS
Sudbury, Massachusetts
BOSTON   TORONTO   LONDON   SINGAPORE

World Headquarters
Jones and Bartlett
Publishers
40 Tall Pine Drive
Sudbury, MA 01776
info@jbpub.com
www.jbpub.com

Jones and Bartlett
Publishers Canada
2406 Nikanna Road
Mississauga, ON L5C
2W6
CANADA

Jones and Bartlett
Publishers International
Barb House, Barb Mews
London W6 7PA
UK

Library of Congress Cataloging-in-Publication Data
McClay, Edward F.
   100 questions & answers about melanoma and other skin cancers / Edward
F. McClay, Mary-Eileen T. McClay, Jodie Smith.
     p. cm.
Includes bibliographical references and index.
 ISBN 0-7637-2036-4
 1. Skin--Cancer--Popular works. 2. Melanoma--Popular works. I.
Title: One hundred questions and answers about melanoma and other skin
cancers. II. McClay, Mary-Eileen T. III. Smith, Jodie. IV. Title.
 RC280.S5M3625 2003
 616.99'477--dc21

                          2002154859

The authors, editor, and publisher have made every effort to provide accurate information.
However, they are not responsible for errors, omissions, or for any outcomes related to the use
of the contents of this book and take no responsibility for the use of the products described.
Treatments and side effects described in this book may not be applicable to all patients; likewise, some patients may require a dose or experience a side effect that is not described herein.
The reader should confer with his or her own physician regarding specific treatments and side
effects. Drugs and medical devices are discussed that may have limited availability controlled by
the Food and Drug Administration (FDA) for use only in a research study or clinical trial. The
drug information presented has been derived from reference sources, recently published data,
and pharmaceutical tests. Research, clinical practice, and government regulations often change
the accepted standard in this field. When consideration is being given to use of any drug in the
clinical setting, the health care provider or reader is responsible for determining FDA status of
the drug, reading the package insert, reviewing prescribing information for the most up-to-
date recommendations on dose, precautions, and contraindications, and determining the
appropriate usage for the product. This is especially important in the case of drugs that are new
or seldom used.

Acquisitions Editor: Christopher Davis
Production Editor: Elizabeth Platt
Cover Design: Philip Regan
Manufacturing Buyer: Therese Bräuer
Composition: Northeast Compositors
Printing and Binding: Malloy Lithographing
Cover Printer: Malloy Lithographing

Printed in the United States of America
07 06 05 04 03   10 9 8 7 6 5 4 3 2 1

Contents

Skin cancer is the most common form of cancer in the United States today. More than 1,000,000 people in the United States will develop non-melanoma skin cancers and another 50,000 individuals will develop malignant melanoma. There are two common types of non-melanoma skin cancer: basal cell carcinoma, which accounts for approximately 700,000 skin cancer cases, and squamous cell carcinoma, which accounts for approximately 300,000 cases. Death from non-melanoma skin cancer is rare. Fewer than 2,500 deaths from non-melanoma skin cancer occur per year.

Malignant melanoma, also known simply as melanoma, is the leading cause of cancer deaths in young women between the ages of 24 and 29. In the year 2002, there will be approximately 7,700 deaths from this disease. In the United States, one person dies each hour from melanoma. The incidence of malignant melanoma has increased by more than 4% each year—faster than any other cancer in the Unites States today. In addition to its rising incidence, malignant melanoma is ranked second on the list of cancers that cause patients to lose the greatest number of years of their productive lives.

This text will provide you with answers to many of the common questions that patients and their families ask about skin cancer. There are several different types of skin cancer, and we will attempt to provide information on the most common forms.

Edward F. McClay, MD
Mary-Eileen T. McClay
Jodie Smith

In the Americas, the earliest cases of melanoma date to pre-Columbian times. Deposits of melanin pigment indicative of metastases have been found in the bones of Inca mummies. However, the disease was and is rare among the native peoples of the Americas. It was not until the early part of the 20th century that the constellation of events began to converge that later resulted in a rapid rise of incidence of cutaneous melanoma. The first was the immigration of large numbers of sun-sensitive Europeans, such as those of Celtic ancestry, to the Americas, particularly to the United States and Canada. The establishment of fair labor practices led to the end of the "sun up to sun down" workday and the advent of leisure time. Clothing for both men and women became less complicated—and skimpier. The ideal of a "peaches and cream" complexion was replaced by the search for the perfect suntan. Ladies with parasols and men with hats gave way to teenagers with Speedos and bikinis. Who among the baby boomers does not remember baby oil and iodine? The net result is that the lifetime risk of developing melanoma for a Caucasian individual born and raised in the United States has now risen to about 1 in 90.

Public Health officials were slow to recognize the deleterious effects of the sun. And as with other health-preserving lifestyle recommendations (such as smoking cessation), the public has been slow to adopt sun-sense advice. However, the media have done an excellent job in educating the public to the dangers of the sun's ultraviolet rays and in increasing public awareness of the early signs of cutaneous melanoma and other skin cancers. Indeed, I believe that the media have been more successful in educating the public than the health care professions have been in educating their members. Continuing medical education is a licensure requirement in virtually all jurisdictions, and I have given and attended hundreds of CME lectures. In one two-week period, I gave the same talk at two different hospitals in the same city. At my second talk, I recognized an attendee from the earlier presentation and became concerned that there were points that I was not making clear. On questioning, however, the individual admitted that he actually wasn't paying much attention, but attended for the free lunch and to socialize with his colleagues.

100 Questions & Answers About Melanoma and Other Skin Cancers presents the relevant information in more detail than is possible in a sound bite, and more cogently than in the usual mass-market material written for consumption by a lay audience. This results from the joint authorship of an experienced and skilled educator (Mary-Eileen T. McClay) and a physician who has dedicated his professional career to the diagnosis and treatment of melanoma (Edward F. McClay, MD). There are alternative sources for information on the effects of sunlight and the signs of skin cancer. The advice provided by the McClays is refined by 20 years of experience dealing with the problem. For example, the McClays counsel that sunscreens are not merely a harmless preventive measure, but rather a third line of defense after common sense and clothing. Further, they advise that there is little added benefit to using a product with an SPF greater than 20 as the additional protection does not justify the increased chemical exposure.

The individuals for whom this book will be of greatest value are those who are newly diagnosed with skin cancer, especially melanoma, and those who have experienced a recurrence of their disease. Jodie's comment on p. 64 is typical of the emotions experienced by a patient when first diagnosed. Quite often, like Jodie, the patients are young, planning their futures, and not pondering their mortality. Traditionally, such patients have relied on their dermatologist, surgeon, or medical oncologist for education and advice. This is a heterogeneous group of health care providers with increasingly limited time and variable experience with the disease that have not had the opportunity to hone their clinical and educational skills with many hundreds of patients, each with individual needs. The patient must be advised not only of the recommended treatment, but also how this treatment fits into his or her life. For example, high dose interferon is the Food and Drug Administration–approved adjuvant treatment following surgery in patients with regional lymph node disease, yet the cost/benefit ratio may not be favorable for all patients. The McClays present a lucid, experience-based, and unbiased discussion of the issue. The Appendix to this book provides a valuable listing of available resources, and the Glossary is a ready reference for lay definitions of medical terms.

Knowledge empowers the patient to make the right choices and to accept the consequences of their circumstance.

Michael J. Mastrangelo, MD
Director, Melanoma Program
Kimmel Cancer Center
Thomas Jefferson University
Philadelphia, PA

PART ONE

The Basics

What is skin?

What is cancer?

What are normal moles? Are they different from freckles?

More . . .

1. What is skin?

Believe it or not, the skin is the largest organ in the body. It's technically called the **integument**. The integument consists of the skin, nails, hair, and all of the different types of **glands**. Skin covers us from head to toe, protecting us from injury by substances in our environment. It also helps to regulate our body temperature, excretes water and other substances, and is an extremely important organ of the senses. The skin is able to sense touch, temperature, and pain.

Skin is composed of two different layers: the **epidermis** and the **dermis** (Figure 1). The epidermis is the outer layer of the skin that is visible to our eyes. The dermis is underneath the epidermis. The epidermis varies in thickness depending on which part of the body it covers. For example, the epidermis is typically thinner over the arm than when it covers an area commonly subjected to increased pressure, such as the soles

Integument

The largest organ of the body composed of the skin and all of its accessory organs, such as hair follicles, nerves, and glands.

Gland

A collection of cells that produces and releases a substance that is used elsewhere in the body, such as a sweat gland.

Epidermis

The outer layer of the skin that forms our first line of protection against harmful elements in our environment.

Dermis

The layer of the skin that underlies the epidermis.

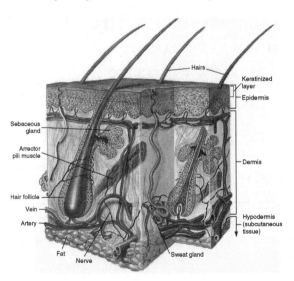

Figure 1.   The structure of human skin. (Reproduced from Alters S, Biology: Understanding Life. Copyright © 2000 by Jones and Bartlett Publishers, Inc., Sudbury, MA).

of the feet. The epidermis is composed primarily of **basal** and **squamous cells**. Each day, your body must replace skin cells that are lost due to normal activity. The new cells are generated at the base of the epidermis by the basal cells. Basal cells are usually tall, thin, and shaped like small columns. These cells form the lowest layer of the epidermis and are the source for cells that will eventually become squamous cells. The basal cells reproduce themselves constantly and are packed together tightly. However, as more and more basal cells are formed, there is not enough room for new cells. Therefore, some of the basal cells are pushed upwards. As the basal cells move upwards they begin to flatten out, ultimately going from a tall thin cell to a flat elongated cell called a squamous cell.

As the squamous cells are pushed closer to the surface of the skin, they become so flat that their **nucleus** is pushed out from the cell. Squamous cells are packed tightly together to form a thick layer, called the cornified layer, in which it becomes impossible to see individual cells under a microscope. This process happens to a greater or lesser degree depending on the area of the skin involved. For instance, the skin over the back of the hand is thin and the cornified layer of cells is not well developed. However, on the surface of the palm this layer is very thick, especially in individuals who perform manual labor.

Melanocytes are specialized cells that make a pigment called **melanin**. The majority of melanocytes are found in the skin but they are also found in special parts of the brain and eyes as well as in the linings of the mouth, vagina, and rectum. Melanocytes in the skin can be found among the basal cells in the lowest layer of the epidermis.

Basal cells

Cells found in the lowest layer of the epidermis of the skin that do not make the protein keratin.

Squamous cells

Cells that are found in the epidermis that are flat and elongated. They are formed from the lower or basal cells of the skin that are shaped like columns and flatten out as they are pushed towards the surface of the skin.

Nucleus

The structure within a cell that contains the DNA. It is usually identifiable under a microscope.

Melanocytes

Cells that make a pigment called melanin.

Melanin

A dark brown pigment made in small granules called melanosomes, within the melanocyte.

The Basics

The dermis is found below the epidermis and is composed primarily of connective **tissue**. It's generally divided into two different layers: the **papillary** and **reticular layers**. The papillary layer is directly below the epidermis and is composed of fine connective tissue fibers that help give structure to the skin. Deeper into the dermis, the connective tissue fibers become larger and thicker. This area is the reticular layer. The dermis is rich with blood and **lymphatic vessels**—an important point to remember when the development of malignant melanoma is discussed. Below the dermis is subcutaneous tissue that contains various accessory organs such as glands for sweating, hair follicles, blood and lymphatic vessels, and nerves.

2. *What is cancer?*

To answer this question, it's necessary to review some basic biology and define a few important concepts: cells, DNA, and mutations. The **cell** is called the basic unit of life because it's the smallest increment that can truly be alive and can reproduce itself. The association of approximately ten billion different individual cells forms the human body. Each cell works with other cells to form the different organs of the body that perform a variety of functions. Cells originate from the union of the sperm and egg, which join to form the first cell of any individual. This first cell undergoes a process called **mitosis** or cell division, which forms a second cell. Each of these two cells can now divide and produce additional cells. This process is repeated many times before a complete baby is formed.

Tissue

The collection of similar cell types that form together to provide a specific function in the body, such as heart muscle cells.

Papillary layer

The first layer beneath the dermis. It typically contains collagen and accessory organs of the skin.

Reticular layer

The reticular layer of the skin is located between the papillary layer and the subcutaneous layer. It is composed primarily of reticulin and collagen fibers that provide a supporting function for the skin.

Lymphatic vessel

A tube-like structure in the body that carries lymphatic fluid through lymph nodes and back to the blood stream.

Cell

The basic unit of life; the smallest component of the body that can independently reproduce itself.

A cell is normally comprised of a **cell membrane** that contains **cytoplasm** and a nucleus, which is where the cell's **DNA** (deoxyribonucleic acid) is found. When the cell is not attempting to divide, the nucleus contains DNA in its **chromatin** state—that is, unwound and in the form of long strands loosely floating in the matrix material of the nucleus. However, when the cell is going to divide, it must double the amount of DNA and then condense this material into the form of **chromosomes**, which are then distributed evenly to each "offspring" cell.

DNA is the genetic material that contains the code responsible for every action that occurs within a cell. It's composed of a long series of connected chemicals or molecules called **nucleic acids**. There are four different nucleic acids found in DNA: adenine (A), guanine (G), cytosine (C), and thymine (T). The nucleic acids are connected to a sugar called deoxyribose and a chemical called phosphoric acid, which helps to provide energy for the various chemical reactions that these molecules undergo. The molecules are then chemically bonded together to form a very long chain. Such a chain might contain the short sequence of adenine, guanine, guanine, cytosine, thymine, cytosine, adenine, cytosine, guanine, thymine, and cytosine. This chain is diagrammed as AGGCTCACGTC. However, these few letters represent only a short part of an entire DNA sequence; there usually are hundreds of thousands of nucleic acids in any one chain.

Mitosis

The name given to the process of cell division that skin cells undergo on a continuous basis.

Cell membrane

A thin envelope composed of lipids and proteins responsible for maintaining cellular structure.

Cytoplasm

The matrix material in a cell that provides the internal location for many activities required for normal function.

DNA (deoxyribonucleic acid)

A double-stranded chain of chemicals that are found in the nucleus of a cell.

Chromatin

A network of fine strands of DNA that is dispersed within the matrix of the nucleus.

Chromosome

DNA that has been condensed and compacted into a structure that is visible under the microscope.

The Basics

Nucleic acids

The class of chemicals that make up the base pairs in the DNA chain.

The nucleic acids in this chain are highly energized and like to attach to each other. Because of their structure, nucleic acids have a very specific binding pattern. Adenosine binds only to thymine and guanine binds only to cytosine. As one long chain is formed by nucleic acids, a second chain attaches to it. These two chains then undergo chemical reactions to form a spring-like structure called a double helix. Using the sequence shown above, the two chains would have the following sequence:

GAATCTGTACT

CTTAGACATGA

This nucleic acid chain provides the basis for the genetic code. The sequence of nucleic acids is read by a special set of chemicals in the cell's nucleus and ultimately transcribes into a variety of different **proteins**. Cells use proteins to perform the many functions necessary for them to survive and carry on their normal activities. The region of DNA that codes for a particular protein is referred to as a **gene**. Genes, which you inherit from your parents, make you who you are and determine what you look like.

Protein

A chain of chemicals composed of amino acids that are linked to one another that participate in many of the body's normal functions.

Gene

A specific sequence of DNA that the cell can read and that results in the production of a protein. Genes are inherited from our parents.

Cancer

The uncontrolled growth of a certain type of cell.

So what does all of this have to do with cancer? Well, simply stated, **cancer** is a condition in which there is uncontrolled growth of a particular type of cell. Cell reproduction continues even when your body has no apparent need for the additional cells.

How does this uncontrolled growth come about? It can occur in one of two ways: either through an error in copying of a DNA sequence during cell division, or through faulty repair of damaged DNA. There are a number of chemical or environmental factors, such as **ultraviolet (UV) radiation**, that can break the DNA chain or cause it to kink in an abnormal fashion. Repair **enzymes** usually repair the break or kink, but these enzymes occasionally make mistakes. Such mistakes in duplicating DNA are called **mutations**. A mutation is a change in the DNA's original sequence. For example, the sequence ATTCG may change to ATCCG, meaning that the second instance of thymine in the DNA chain has been changed to a cytosine. This simple change in the sequence may change the protein that is produced, thus making the protein inactive. If a protein's original function was to help control the growth of the cell, a mutation may give the cell an advantage over other cells, potentially causing a malignant cell. In some cases the change in the sequence may make the new cell stronger in some fashion. In other cases, the change may be lethal and the new cell will die.

It's generally believed that most cancers begin from a single cell through a process called **initiation**. A variety of different biologic events can initiate damage to DNA resulting in the development of the cancer cell. An accumulation of genetic mutations in the cancer cell ultimately gives it a growth advantage over other cells in the area. This accumulation of genetic mutations occurs through a process called **promotion**. Promotion may be the result of another agent acting upon the cancer cell and its environment to continue to provide this abnormal cell with growth advantage. Another name for a cancer cell is a **malignant cell**. A

The Basics

Ultraviolet (UV) radiation

Electromagnetic radiation from the sun that is responsible for sun induced damage to the skin.

Enzymes

Proteins that function in the body to increase the rate at which these chemical reactions occur.

Mutation

Any change in the sequence of base pairs in the DNA chain.

Initiation

The initial insult to a gene that leads to a malignant cell or cancer.

Promotion

A factor that stimulates the growth of malignant cells, providing a stimulus that enhances survival and reproduction.

Malignant cell

A cell that has accumulated abnormalities in its genetic makeup that give it a growth advantage.

hallmark of malignant cells is the continued accumulation of genetic mutations until the death of the patient.

Cancer cells are resilient and able to tolerate a variety of hostile attacks against them. This is what makes it so difficult to treat cancer. In many cases the treatment works in some of the cells and not others. In this situation, the patient commonly experiences a decrease in the size of **tumors**, only to have them grow back in greater number. As the tumors begin to take over normal organs, they compromise the function of these organs, ultimately resulting in the patient's death.

Another feature of cancer cells is their ability to break off from the **primary site** (the original location where the cancer started) and to travel to different areas of the body, a process called **metastasis**. These cells can enter the blood stream or the **lymph fluid,** which travel throughout the body. The cells then exit the fluid and migrate into the surrounding tissue. Common sights of metastasis include the **lymph nodes**, the lung, the liver, bones, and the brain. Certain malignancies have a tendency to metastasize to specific organs but melanomas have a reputation of spreading to just about any area of the body. This process involves many changes to the cells that allow them to survive in the blood's hostile environment and then escape into another organ. Once they establish themselves in the new organ, the malignant cells begin to grow and invade the organ, causing substantial damage to the body. Without effective treatment, the growth of malignant cells will continue, ultimately causing death.

Tumor

A disordered growth of cells that result in a collection of like cells commonly forming a nodule or lump. A tumor can be benign (non-cancerous) or malignant (cancer).

Primary site

The site where a cancer begins; where the first cancer cell was formed.

Metastasis

The process by which a cancer cell leaves the area where it originated and begins to grow in a new part of the body.

Lymph fluid

Fluid that normally leaks out of the blood and collects in tissue.

3. What are normal moles? Are they different from freckles?

Normal **moles** usually begin as small (1 to 3 mm), pigmented **lesions** that appear on a sun-exposed surface of skin. Such moles usually appear early in childhood and are termed **junctional moles** or **nevi**. Moles are structures in the skin that are composed primarily of nevus cells and melanocytes, and they have a cellular structure that can be identified by examination under a microscope. Moles are found on the skin of essentially every individual and are usually of no consequence. They can appear anywhere on the skin, either alone or in groups, typically numbering between 30 and 40. Typically found on skin surfaces that are exposed to the sun, moles tend to be dark in color (usually some shade of brown); however, moles can be flesh colored. Moles vary in size and shape and sometimes grow thick, coarse hairs.

A child born with a mole is considered to have a **congenital mole.** This occurs in approximately 1 out of 100 births. As individuals age, new moles appear, and those that are already present begin to change. Moles can vary in size and shape throughout their lifetime but most will be less than 6 mm—about the size of a pencil eraser. When they grow and elevate off of the skin's surface they are called **compound moles**. Towards the end of their natural history, moles may lose their pigment and become flesh colored. These are called **dermal moles**. This process takes about 50 years, and ultimately leads to the complete disappearance of the mole.

The Basics

Lymph node

A small, typically round or oval nodule that is comprised of millions of immune cells called lymphocytes and found in many areas of the body.

Mole

An appendage of the skin that includes a collection of nevus cells and melanocytes.

Lesion

An abnormal structure on the skin that is either benign or malignant.

Junctional mole

The earliest form of a mole where the cells develop at the junction of the dermis with the epidermis.

Nevus, nevi

Another name for a mole.

Congenital mole

A mole that is present at birth, ranging in size from a few millimeters to bathing suit size.

In very rare situations children are born with a large congenital mole called a **bathing suit nevus**. In this situation, the mole occupies a large portion of the child's body, often involving the trunk of the body. This type of mole can be quite disfiguring, presenting a variety of problems for the child.

Freckles don't have cellular structure. They are simply areas of the skin that have a higher amount of pigment. Freckles are usually well circumscribed and vary from light tan to dark brown. They will frequently darken in the summer after sun exposure, and tend to fade in the winter months. There is no risk of the freckle itself becoming malignant.

4. I have heard the term dysplastic mole. What does this mean?

There is a variant of a normal mole that is called a **dysplastic mole**. Dysplastic moles are not malignant in and of themselves, but they have been associated with the development of malignant melanoma. Dysplastic moles are usually bigger than normal moles with irregular shapes and multiple colors (Plate 1). They can occur in any part of the body but are most commonly found in sun-exposed areas. In most cases, the diagnosis can be made by examining the mole clinically; however, sometimes the diagnosis can only be made by a **biopsy** (see Questions 32, 34, and 36 for more about biopsies). The dysplastic mole looks different under a microscope compared to a normal mole; it has more abnormal melanocytes and is populated with immune cells.

Sometimes melanoma actually develops in the dysplastic mole, but in many cases the dysplastic mole serves as a marker to identify individuals who have an increased risk of a melanoma somewhere else on the skin. In rare cases, the melanoma is part of a syndrome called the dysplastic nevus (or mole) syndrome. Children or adolescents with this syndrome begin to develop dysplastic moles around the age of puberty. Individuals with the most severe form of this syndrome who develop dysplastic moles ultimately develop melanoma sometime during their lifetime. These individuals are likely to develop multiple melanomas and must be followed for their entire life by having a health care professional perform skin examinations at least twice a year. If an individual has many moles, more frequent examinations may be warranted. Investigators are developing imaging systems that will store pictures of patients' skin so that there is a permanent record against which to compare subsequent skin examinations.

Another type of pigmented lesion on the skin is called **seborrheic keratosis**. Seborrheic keratosis is a **benign** lesion of the skin that sometimes mimics melanoma. This lesion is the result of progressive growth of normal cells in the skin. It tends to be a thick, raised, pigmented lesion that appears as if it has been pasted onto the skin. Cases of seborrheic keratosis are common in the middle aged and the elderly, and are typically

The Basics

Biopsy

The surgical removal and microscopic examination of tissue from the body for the purpose of establishing a precise diagnosis.

Seborrheic keratosis

A benign skin lesion common in older individuals. These lesions typically appear as thick, yellow, waxy growths that look as if they have been "stuck" onto the skin.

Benign

A biologic state of abnormal growth of cells that are not cancer cells, i.e., they have no potential to spread throughout the body.

found in sun-exposed areas. Seborrheic keratosis isn't cancerous and isn't likely to develop into any sort of skin cancer. If you have seborrheic keratosis, you shouldn't worry about it turning into melanoma.

5. What is skin cancer? What causes it?

Cancer is typically named for the type of cell from which the cancer originated, the organ where the cancer started, or both. For instance, squamous cell carcinoma derives from squamous cells, but can originate in either the skin or in the esophagus. If the cancer originates in the skin, it's referred to as skin cancer, if the cancer originates in the esophagus it's called esophageal cancer—but both are forms of squamous cell cancers. Therefore, skin cancer is cancer that begins in the skin. As described above, there are a variety of cells in the skin that can become malignant or cancerous. It's estimated that there are more than 1 million new cases of skin cancer in the United States each year.

Most skin cancer can be prevented by limiting the skin's exposure to sunlight.

Most skin cancers are the result of damage to the genetic information contained in the nucleus of a cell in the skin—damage caused primarily by UV rays from the sun. This factor is discussed extensively in Part 2. Although there are some factors that can predispose a person to skin cancer (see Question 7), most skin cancer can be prevented by limiting the skin's exposure to sunlight.

6. *What are the different kinds of skin cancer?*

As mentioned in the introduction, there are three basic forms of skin cancer: basal cell carcinoma, squamous cell carcinoma, and malignant melanoma. **Basal cell carcinoma** is a cancer of the skin that develops from the basal cells of the skin. These cells are in the deepest layer of the skin and are the source of cells that become squamous cells as they migrate to the surface of the skin. Basal cell carcinoma is the most common cancer in the United States, accounting for more than 80% of all skin cancers. Last year approximately 900,000 new cases were diagnosed. Despite the very large number of patients who develop basal cell carcinoma, it's an extremely uncommon cause of cancer deaths. Once it develops, this cancer tends to grow and invade locally at a very slow rate. Left on the skin, basal cell carcinomas will invade local tissue over the course of many years, rarely metastasizing to another organ. Basal cell carcinomas can become very destructive locally if not addressed early enough. Early diagnosis is very important. The reconstructive surgery that might be necessary to correct the defect resulting from removing a basal cell carcinoma can be extensive because these lesions will invade underlying structures while the overlying skin appears normal.

These lesions occur commonly on the face and upper extremities. They usually begin as an area of raised, red tissue with a pearly texture that shines in the light

Basal cell carcinoma

A malignant tumor that arises in the basal cells of the epidermis. Basal cell carcinoma can be locally invasive, but seldom metastasizes.

Basal cell carcinoma is an extremely uncommon cause of cancer deaths.

(Plate 2). They commonly have small blood vessels in them that will sometimes break, resulting in visible blood within the lesion.

Squamous cell carcinoma

A cancer of the cells in the skin called squamous cells. This cancer is usually curable, however, in some patients, especially those with immune deficiencies, it can be lethal.

Ulceration

The loss of the most superficial layer of the epidermis that results in an inflammatory reaction in the skin or tumor.

The ability to metastasize distinguishes melanoma from the other skin cancers.

Mucosal surface

The lining surface of any one of the many internal areas of the body such as mouth, esophagus, vagina, or rectum.

Accounting for more than 200,000 cases of skin cancer in 1998, **squamous cell carcinoma** is the second most common form of the disease, representing 16% of all skin cancers. Like basal cell carcinoma, this disease is 95% curable if it's caught early. But squamous cell carcinoma can spread—and is potentially lethal—if left untreated. Squamous cell carcinoma typically begins as a hard, crusting, scaling patch, and commonly has a central **ulcer** (Plate 3). The edges of the lesion are usually red with raised borders surrounding the ulcer. They also are most common on skin surfaces that are exposed to the sun.

As mentioned above, malignant melanoma is a cancer of the melanocytes, the cells that are responsible for the production of melanin. Melanoma is the third most common form of skin cancer, but is responsible for most of the deaths related to skin cancer. Unlike basal and squamous cell cancers that tend to invade locally, melanoma will quickly find a way to spread to other parts of the body. It's this ability to metastasize that distinguishes melanoma from the other skin cancers.

Melanoma typically begins on sun-exposed surfaces of the skin, but in rare cases it can develop on a **mucosal surface** such as the mouth, rectum, or vagina. Lesions are usually pigmented, appearing in a shade of brown or black (Plate 4). About 10% of patients will have **amelanotic** lesions. Such lesions are flesh colored.

There are other forms of cancer that begin in the skin, such as Merkel cell carcinoma, Kaposi's sarcoma, and some forms of lymphoma; however, these cancers are quite rare. They will be discussed briefly at the end of this book.

Amelanotic

A melanoma that doesn't make pigment; typically red or pink in color instead of brown or black.

The Basics

15

PART TWO

Risk Factors

Who is at risk for developing skin cancer?

What gives skin its color? How do we tan?

Who is at risk to develop malignant melanoma?

More ...

PERSONAL FACTORS

7. Who is at risk for developing skin cancer?

As a general rule, individuals who have pale skin, red or blonde hair, blue, green, or gray eyes, sensitivity to UV radiation (relative inability to tan), and tendency to freckle or form pigmented moles are most at risk to develop skin cancer. These individuals absorb more UV radiation per unit time than an individual who has naturally darker skin. Within the white population there is an increased incidence of skin cancer among those individuals with lighter skin. For example, individuals of Irish descent with pale skin who tan poorly are at higher risk than individuals of Italian descent with darker skin who tan well. Those individuals who have a natural tan and who don't burn and only darken their skin in the sun are at least risk. Despite this, many individuals with dark skin develop skin cancer, and many have died from malignant melanoma.

Less risk does not mean no risk.

As a general rule of thumb, the darker your skin is, the less risk you have of developing skin cancer—but less risk does not mean *no* risk. Although it's true that most people who get skin cancer have light skin, individuals with dark skin occasionally develop malignant skin lesions. In particular, dark-skinned individuals must be concerned about any changing mole. Malignant melanoma in dark-skinned individuals tends to develop in areas of skin that are less pigmented. Therefore, a changing lesion on the palms of the hands, on the soles of the feet, or underneath the fingernails should cause particular concern.

In some families or individuals, there is a genetic pre-disposition to developing skin cancer that goes beyond skin color. For instance, individuals with a disease called xeroderma pigmentosa have defective DNA repair mechanisms that allow UV-induced damage to remain as part of the normal genetic makeup of the cell. Over time, the mutations accumulate, ultimately causing skin cancer. In particular, these individuals are at risk for developing squamous cell carcinomas that carry a higher risk of spreading.

Additionally, individuals who have a defective immune system, such as those with acquired immunodeficiency syndrome (AIDS), lymphomas, or those on immuno-suppressive medications after undergoing an organ transplant have a 4-fold to 5-fold increase in skin cancer. Finally, individuals who have a high number of abnormal moles are at increased risk for developing melanoma.

Children who are born with moles are said to have con-genital moles (see Question 3). As a general rule, congenital moles are not necessarily associated with the development of skin cancer. However, large congenital moles have been associated with a tendency to turn into malignant melanoma. As the size of the congenital mole increases, so does the risk of developing melanoma. Congenital moles that are greater than 5 cm in diameter should be observed carefully. If an area of the mole begins to change, a physician should evaluate the mole.

In general, children with a large number of freckles are children who tan poorly and sunburn easily, putting them at higher risk for skin cancer. Thus, freckles are indirectly associated with developing skin cancer.

Sunscreen

An agent that, when applied to the skin, provides a chemical barrier, absorbing UV radiation before it can enter deeper layers of the skin.

Studies show that children with freckles are especially in need of **sunscreen**. In a recent study conducted in Vancouver, British Columbia, Dr. David McLean found 30% to 40% fewer new moles on freckled children using sunscreen than freckled children not using sunscreen. Because moles and freckles together may put a person at greater risk for developing a skin cancer, using sunscreen is even more important.

8. What gives skin its color? How do we tan?

Eumelanin

The chemical form of melanin that is responsible for brown/black coloration of the skin.

Phaeomelanin

The chemical form of melanin that is responsible for red/yellow coloration.

Skin coloration is genetically determined at birth. Pigments in the skin produce its color. Skin color varies depending on the type of pigments present and the amount of pigment that is produced. Melanin is the major pigment produced by melanocytes. It's produced in two forms: **eumelanin**, which creates a brown-black coloration, and **phaeomelanin**, which produces yellow-red coloration. Once melanin is produced, it's released from the melanocyte and absorbed by other cells in the skin, primarily the squamous cells. As the melanin is dispersed in the squamous cells, the skin takes on a brown-black or yellow-red coloration depending upon the predominant form of melanin that's produced. This process creates your normal skin color (also called your constitutive skin color).

Melanin production varies depending on a person's racial or ethnic background. Essentially, everyone has the same number of melanocytes. What's different in individuals is the type and amount of melanin that the melanocytes produce. For example, those of Celtic origin tend to produce very little melanin compared with those of Italian descent. Individuals of African descent usually produce a tremendous amount of eumelanin, the form of melanin that makes skin a brown-black color. Individuals of Asian descent produce more phaeomelanin, which results in skin that is a yellow-red color.

When your skin is exposed to UV radiation from the sun, the melanocytes are stimulated to increase in number as well as increase production of melanin. This process is referred to as tanning. Depending on a variety of genetic factors, some individuals tan very well and others hardly tan at all. Intense accumulations of melanin will turn the skin dark in color. Less production of melanin may not even be recognizable. Melanin has the ability to absorb the sun's damaging UV radiation, thus preventing it from reaching the deeper layers of the skin where it damages important cellular structures.

9. I have psoriasis and I'm currently receiving PUVA treatments. Does this put me at higher risk to develop skin cancer?

Recent studies have demonstrated that patients who undergo PUVA treatment are at increased risk to develop both melanoma and non-melanoma skin cancer. This risk must now be taken into account when making the decision regarding this form of treatment. You should discuss this risk with your physician and determine how to best minimize your risk. Additionally, you and your physician should agree to a regular skin check schedule so that any skin cancers that might develop will be diagnosed early.

10. Who is at risk to develop malignant melanoma?

Jodie's comment:

I was so uneducated about any type of skin cancer. Certainly, I had no idea that you could die from it. I would never want to mislead anyone to thinking that you need to be quite fair in color. While certainly individuals with fair skin are at increased risk, I have a friend who is Hispanic who developed melanoma. Her melanoma is on her thigh. I understand that the bottom of the feet and under the fingernails is also a target for any of us but is more common in individuals with dark skin.

In general, those patients who are at risk for developing skin cancer include those at risk for melanoma. However, there are additional circumstances that favor the development of melanoma. They include:

- individuals with a history of sunburns before the age of 15
- individuals with a family history of malignant melanoma
- individuals with dysplastic moles
- individuals with a personal history of having a prior melanoma; these individuals have a 3% to 5% chance of developing a second melanoma
- individuals with disorders of their immune system, such as organ transplant patients, AIDS patients, or patients with a history of lymphoma.

Although everyone should be aware of changes in moles, if you have any of the above risk factors and you notice a change in a mole, you should visit your physician as soon as possible for an evaluation.

ENVIRONMENTAL RISK FACTORS

11. What environmental factors are important?

We are all aware that we should use sunscreen on bright sunny days, but we can be exposed to significant amounts of UV radiation even on cloudy days. It's estimated that 85% of the total UV radiation reaches the Earth's surface on a cloudy day. Therefore, we must pay particular attention to protecting ourselves every day. Other environmental factors to keep in mind include the reflection of UV radiation off of a variety of surfaces. In particular, water, snow, and light-colored concrete surfaces reflect significant amounts of UV radiation. These factors must be taken into account when you prepare your protective regimen. For example, if you're planning a day at the beach, you must still put on sunscreen to prevent the damage that will occur as a result of indirect reflection of the UV radiation—even if you plan to spend the majority of the day under a large umbrella. Similarly, using a sunscreen is an important part of protection during snow or water skiing because both of these surfaces will reflect UV radiation.

We must pay particular attention to protecting ourselves every day.

12. What is UV radiation? What is meant by UVA, UVB, and UVC?

The sun provides the Earth with energy primarily in the form of light, heat, radio waves, and other components of what's referred to as the electromagnetic spectrum. This energy travels to the Earth in wave-like patterns, which can be described in terms of the waves' length and frequency. Energy with the shortest wavelength and highest frequency reaches the Earth in the form of UV and gamma rays. There are three recog nized spectrums of UV rays that are based on wavelengths and frequency. These spectrums are referred to as UVA, UVB, and UVC. UVA has the longest wavelength and lowest frequency while UVC has the shortest wavelength and highest frequency.

UVA radiation remains relatively constant throughout the year. It's also the most common form of UV radiation emitted from tanning booth bulbs. UVA, because of its long wavelength, penetrates deep into the layers of the skin and is thought to be the spectrum most responsible for wrinkling of the skin.

Although it remains somewhat controversial, there is evidence to suggest that UVA can function as an initiator of malignant melanoma by causing damage to the DNA, which in turn initiates the cancer. More recent research has shown that UVA radiation is a potent **immunosuppressive agent**. The skin contains many immune cells that help to protect us from a variety of potential problems, including skin cancer. Researchers have recently demonstrated that exposing skin to UVA radiation results in a significant depletion of the skin's immune cells. This depletion of immune cells provides malignant cells with a growth advantage. So, UVA functions as a tumor promoter.

UVB intensity, which is more damaging than UVA, varies. UVB is more intense in the summer months, at higher altitudes, and at latitudes at or close to the equator. For example, Florida receives 150% more UVB radiation than Maine. There is clear evidence that UVB functions as a tumor initiator, causing all forms of skin cancer, including melanoma. UVB also

*Immuno-
suppressive agent*

A compound or element that can prevent or slow down the reaction of the natural immune system.

promotes tumor development by inflicting additional DNA damage to the cancer cell.

UVC is potentially the most damaging of the UV rays. However, because of the Earth's atmosphere and, most importantly, the ozone layer, most UVC rays are absorbed and don't reach the Earth's surface. There remains concern, however, that as the ozone layer is depleted, more UVC radiation will reach the Earth's surface, significantly increasing the risk of all forms of skin cancer.

Harmful UV rays are more intense in the summer, at higher altitudes, and closer to the equator. Wind and reflections from water, sand, and snow also increase the sun's harmful effects. Even on cloudy days UV radiation reaches the earth and can cause skin damage. The UV index is a prediction of ultraviolet intensity in a given location. It can be found in the weather section of most daily newspapers and on some television weather forecasts.

Harmful UV rays are more intense in the summer, at higher altitudes, and closer to the equator.

13. Are there geophysical factors that increase my risk for developing skin cancer?

The geophysical factors that are most important in the development of skin cancer are, for the most part, related to factors that increase your exposure to UV radiation. The latitude at which you live is a major determinant of UV exposure. If you live closer to the equator, you're exposed to more UV radiation per unit time than someone who lives at more northern latitude such as in Canada. Keep in mind that the earth is a sphere, so its diameter is greatest at the equator. Therefore, land masses located close to the equator are physically closer to the sun; hence they receive more UV radiation.

Similarly, people who live at higher altitudes, such as in the mountains, also receive greater amounts of UV radiation than those living closer to sea level. Recent studies have shown that the UVB levels in Vail, Colorado—located 8,500 feet above sea level—are 60% higher than those in New York at sea level, and similar to the UVB levels measured in Orlando, Florida, a city 775 miles closer to the equator than Vail. A person with average complexion skiing at 11,000 feet in Vail will receive enough UVB radiation at noon to sunburn after only 6 minutes of unprotected exposure. A similar individual could spend 25 minutes in the sun at noon at sea level before equivalent sunburn would develop.

The time of day also plays an important role in exposure to UV radiation. As the Earth spins on its axis, areas on its surface that are exposed to the sun between the hours of 10 A.M. and 3 P.M. receive the highest amount of UV radiation. In this case the sun is directly overhead, thus the radiation travels to the Earth's surface by the most direct path; the atmosphere deflects less radiation.

The seasons also affect how much UV radiation reaches the Earth's surface. As the earth rotates around the sun, it tilts on its axis. From June until August, such tilting positions countries located in the Northern Hemisphere closer to the sun. During these summer months the amount of UV radiation that people living in the Northern Hemisphere are exposed to increases.

The number of hours the region is exposed to UV radiation also increases.

14. I have heard that pollution may protect us. Is this true?

Air pollution may actually have one beneficial effect. It may deflect UV radiation, providing a modest covering for the surface of the Earth. Although in this one instance pollution seems to be of benefit, the damage it causes to the ozone layer is far more costly and exceeds its minimal protective effect. Ozone is a chemical compound that is concentrated high in the atmosphere and that forms a protective barrier against UV radiation. Current measurements suggest that UVC, the form of UV radiation that carries the most energy (and is potentially the most damaging), doesn't reach the Earth's surface because it's absorbed by the ozone layer. Chemical pollutants such as chlorofluorocarbons that are released in propellants and burning fossil fuels bind to and destroy ozone. As the ozone layer is destroyed, more UVC will reach the Earth's surface, significantly increasing the health risks of many forms of life. It's estimated that for each 10% decrease in the ozone layer there will be a 30% increase in squamous cell cancers, a 50% increase in basal cell cancers, and a 10% increase in malignant melanoma. This will result in a significant increase in the incidence of and mortality associated with these diseases as well as increased health care expenses.

15. What about fluorescent lights? I've heard that they can cause skin cancer.

Fluorescent lights do emit a small amount of UV radiation. However, at this time there is no convincing evidence that they contribute to the skin cancer problem.

There is no convincing evidence that fluorescent lights contribute to the skin cancer problem.

Remember, your skin *does* have a certain amount of natural protection against UV, and sitting indoors under a fluorescent light exposes you to far less UV than you would be exposed to outdoors during daylight—and much less than your skin is normally able to handle without becoming damaged.

16. What is the Ultraviolet index?

In an attempt to provide guidelines for our behavior in the sun, the National Weather Service and the Environmental Protection Agency have developed a scale ranging from 0 to 10+ to estimate the amount of exposure to UV radiation. This UV index (Table 1) is issued daily and provides the next days estimated amount of exposure to UV radiation.

Special care should be taken when the UV index predicts exposure levels of moderate or higher. Avoid deliberate excessive exposure to the sun, such as sunbathing or spending days at the beach. Wear a wide-brimmed hat when you're out in the sun and wear UV-blocking sunglasses and protective clothing. Most

Table 1.   Ultraviolet index

Index Number	Exposure Level	Time to sun damage
0–2	Minimal	>60 (minutes)
3–4	Low	45
5–6	Moderate	30
7–9	High	15
10+	Very High	<10

importantly, use sunscreen to protect any area of exposed skin.

For more information on the UV index, please visit: *www.cpc.ncep.noaa.gov/products/stratosphere/uv_index/uv_current.html*, or call the EPA Stratospheric Ozone Hotline at 800–296–1996 or the National Weather Service at 301–713–0622.

Risk Factors

PART THREE

Prevention and Protection

What can I do to protect myself from UV damage?

Is it a good idea to prepare for sun exposure by visiting a tanning bed prior to going on vacation?

More ...

17. What can I do to protect myself from UV damage?

Jodie's comment:

Since I developed my melanoma, I do not go in the sun for more than 10 minutes or so without using a sunscreen. And not just any sunscreen. It must have both UVA and UVB protection. That way it provides me with maximum protection. Also, it is important to apply it 20 minutes before going into the sun, and reapply it several times during the day, as it can come off.

There are many steps that you can take to reduce the risk of developing skin cancer.

There are many steps that you can take to reduce the risk of developing skin cancer. The first step is to determine your skin type. This will give you a sense of your basic risk. Next, limit your sun exposure during the day. Wear clothing that is tight knit and a wide brimmed hat to increase your protection. Finally, use a broad-spectrum sunscreen to further decrease your risk. Oh, by the way, don't forget your sunglasses!

18. Is it a good idea to prepare for sun exposure by visiting a tanning bed prior to going on vacation?

Absolutely not! This is one of the most common mistakes that many people make. Current tanning bed facilities are supposed to use light sources that emit UVA radiation. UVA-induced tans are not protective. Keep these points in mind:

- As UVA bulbs age, they emit increasing amounts of UVB radiation. Thus, as the bulbs age, your skin may be significantly damaged by UVB exposure.

- UVA is damaging in and of itself. UVA has been found to be a tumor initiator and promoter (as described in Question 12). Therefore, UVA contributes to the cancer problem.
- UVA radiation inhibits the local immune response of the skin and decreases our first line of defense against a variety of problems.
- UVA radiation penetrates into the deeper layers of the epidermis and dermis, resulting in destruction of **collagen** and **elastin fibers**. This results in premature aging (wrinkling) of the skin.

Collagen fibers

A thick fiber that acts to provide strength to a tissue.

Elastin fibers

Fibers that allow a tissue to be flexible yet retain its' natural shape.

Overall, the UVA-induced tan from a tanning bed is less protective than a UVB-induced tan. Microscopic examination of skin that has been tanned as a result of UVA exposure reveals gaping holes in the protective tanning layer. These holes allow UVB radiation to reach the deeper layers of the epidermis without obstruction. Thus, a tan from a tanning bed looks good, but it's minimally protective. Don't subject yourself to this potentially harmful experience.

A tan from a tanning bed looks good, but it's minimally protective.

Government agencies such as the Food and Drug Administration (FDA) and the Centers for Disease Control and Prevention (CDC) have also issued warnings to people to avoid use of tanning beds and sun lamps. The FDA will provide a fact sheet on the hazards of indoor tanning from the FDA's Facts on Demand system by calling 1–800–899–0381 following the voice instructions (select 2 and then Division of Device User Programs and Systems Analysis or DDUPSA; the information will be faxed to you on the same day). This information is also available through the FDA's Web site at *www.fda.gov*. Similar information is available through the American Academy of Dermatology's (AAD's) Web site at *www.aad.org*.

19. What is meant by skin type? What difference does skin type make in the need for UV protection?

Jodie's comment:

Skin type refers to how much natural pigment an individual's skin has without being exposed to the sun. Pigment is important because the more pigment the skin has the more protection it provides—although I would not rely solely on natural pigment for protection. As I said before, even individuals with high levels of natural pigmentation can get melanoma, especially on the bottom of the feet and under the fingernails.

The risk of developing skin cancer is related to the natural protective tanning ability of your skin. The darker your skin is prior to UV exposure, the more natural protection you have. Further, the ability to tan after UV exposure adds to this protection. Table 2 lists skin types as identified by tanning ability.

Table 2. Skin types

Type	Tanning Ability
I. Pale white skin	Always burns; never tans
II. White	Burns easily; tans minimally
III. White (Average)	Burns moderately; tans gradually to light brown
IV. Beige or lightly tanned	Burns minimally; always tans well to moderately brown
V. Moderate brown or tanned	Rarely burns; tans profusely to dark
VI. Dark brown or black	Never burns; deeply pigmented

After using this table to assess your skin type you must then develop a behavior pattern for when you venture out in to the sun. Type I and II individuals are at most risk for UV damage. The risk lessens for darker skin types. This information, along with the UV index, should help you to prepare for your day in the sun.

20. Do I have more protection because I am naturally tanned?

Yes. However, there are several important distinctions to be made regarding an individual's tanning ability. It's important to realize that tanning is the skin's reaction to UV radiation-induced damage. In response to this damage, melanocytes are stimulated to produce melanin, which absorbs even more UV rays. If you already have naturally brown or black skin that is ready to absorb UV radiation, your skin simply gets darker in response to the UV exposure, providing you with the best natural protection.

If you have lighter skin but can tan in response to the UV exposure, you have some degree of natural protection, but you depend on UV damage to initiate the tanning response. Thus, you have to suffer some skin injury to develop the tan. As a result, you're exposing your melanocytes—the cells that have the potential to become the most lethal form of skin cancer—to UV rays to tan your skin. Tanning lighter skin may seem like a good idea at first, but the damage suffered is substantial and must not be discounted. Also, remember that even though a tan does provide some protection, the SPF factor of a tan is only in the range of 3 to 5. You're far better served by protecting yourself from the damage of UV radiation rather than trying to develop a protective tan.

21. What's so important about the time of day?

Time of day as well as the time of year affects the amount of UV radiation that reaches the Earth's surface. As the Earth rotates around the sun it tilts upon its axis of rotation. During the months of December through March, the Earth is tilted in such a way that the Northern Hemisphere is positioned away from the sun, and thus receives less UV exposure. In the Southern Hemisphere, this is the season of highest exposure. Conversely, during the summer months of June to September, the Earth tilts the Northern Hemisphere towards the sun, which makes this area of the Earth receive more UV radiation, while the Southern Hemisphere receives less. Likewise, during the day the rotation of the Earth upon its axis will bring us closer to the sun between the hours of 10 A.M. and 2 P.M. Therefore, during this time there's more UV radiation reaching the surface of the Earth. So, between the hours of 10 A.M. and 2 P.M. we are most at risk to suffer UV injury and must take steps to protect ourselves. This risk is highest during the summer and decreases during the winter.

22. What about clothing? Doesn't that help to protect me from UV radiation?

Clothing can act as a physical block against UV radiation. The tighter the weave of the material, the more protection the material provides. For example, a loose knit shirt that shows some of the underlying skin won't protect you as well as material that is tightly woven.

Not only will this material physically block the sun, but light-colored material will also help to keep the skin cool. A broad-brimmed hat provides additional protection. Keep in mind, however, that the UV protection of material decreases if it becomes wet.

The UV protection of material decreases if it becomes wet.

In response to increased concerns about UV damage and the alarming increase in the rate of melanoma and skin cancers, several manufacturing companies have developed clothing that's given an SPF rating. The clothing has been treated or woven in such a way that as much as 95% of the UV rays are blocked.

23. What is a sunscreen?

Sunscreens are chemical agents that are able to absorb the energy from UV radiation. By applying sunscreen to the skin, UV rays are absorbed before they can enter the skin's layers. There are a wide variety of agents that are able to absorb UV radiation so the ingredients of any given product may vary. They also vary in their effectiveness and potential side effects.

24. What is the difference between a sunscreen and a sunblock?

Typically, sunscreens are considered those agents that, when placed on your skin, interact with UV radiation in a chemical manner, absorbing the energy before it can interact with your DNA. In contrast, **sunblocks** are usually opaque agents that act as a physical barrier to the UV radiation when placed on your skin, reflecting the energy rather than absorbing it. Most sunblocks are thick and visible when placed on the skin.

Sunblock

An agent that, when applied to the skin, provides a physical barrier reflecting UV radiation.

Prevention and Protection

25. My sunscreen has a number, SPF 20, on it. What does this mean?

The term SPF stands for sun protection factor, an indication of how much protection a given product provides. The number is meant to provide a concrete measure of this protection. There are two ways to use this SPF number. The first way involves determining your **minimal erythema dose (MED)**. MED is a measure of how much time given individuals can spend in the sun before they develop a light pink color to their skin (the earliest stage of sunburn). The MED is multiplied by the SPF number of your sunscreen. The resulting number is how much time you can spend in the sun with sunscreen on your skin before turning the same light pink. For example, if you turn light pink within 10 minutes of being exposed to the sun, wearing a sunscreen with an SPF of 10 will allow that you to spend 100 minutes in the sun before you turn the same shade of pink. Thus, the amount of time you can spend in the sun for a given level of UV exposure is increased by a factor of 10.

Minimal erythema dose (MED)

The amount of time it takes for a given individual to turn light pink during sun exposure.

You should also keep in mind that the SPF relates to the absorption of a specific percentage of UV radiation. For instance, using a sunscreen with an SPF of 20 reduces your UV radiation exposure by approximately 98%. If you use anything less than a 20 you begin to lose protection. In contrast, using a product with an SPF of 40 adds very little additional protection.

26. What is PABA?

PABA stands for para-amino benzoic acid, a chemical that was a component of early sunscreens. This compound used to be one of the most effective sunscreen

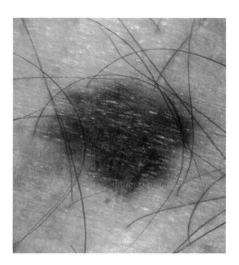

Plate 1. Dysplastic nevus. This type of mole may be a precursor to melanoma. Note the asymmetrical shape with irregular borders and different shades of brown. This particular dysplastic nevus was bigger than a pencil eraser.

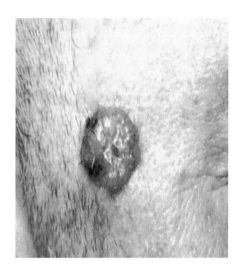

Plate 2. Basal cell carcinoma. These nodular lesions are usually pink or flesh colored. A BCC typically has a "pearly" sheen when light is on it, and you frequently can see small blood vessels in it.

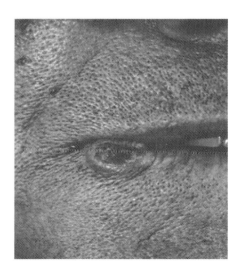

Plate 3. Squamous cell carcinoma. In this instance, the SCC appears as a pink or flesh-colored lesion on the lip that has an ulcer in its center with "heaped up" borders.

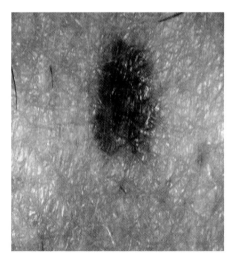

Plate 4. Melanoma in situ. This lesion has an irregular border with several shades of brown and looked similar to the dysplastic nevus. A biopsy was necessary to determine that it was melanoma; the biopsy showed that it had not yet invaded the lower layers of the skin.

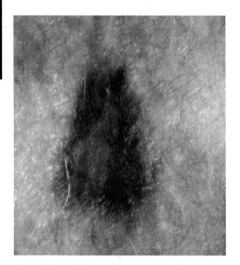

Plate 5. Superficial spreading melanoma. This is the most common type of melanoma. It has an asymmetrical shape with irregular borders and is dark brown to black color; this particular example was approximately 1 cm in diameter.

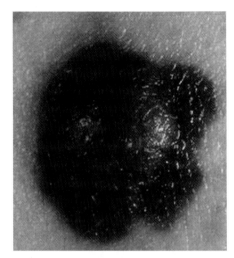

Plate 6. Nodular melanoma. This lesion shows a large nodule growing out of a flat black area on the skin. This form of melanoma invades the skin early in its development.

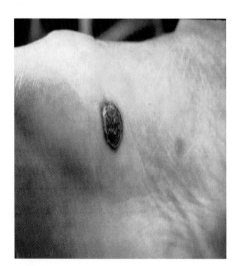

Plate 7. Acral lentigenous mela-noma. Note the black color and scaling of the overlying layers of skin. Its appearance in the sole of the foot classifies it as an acral lentigenous melanoma.

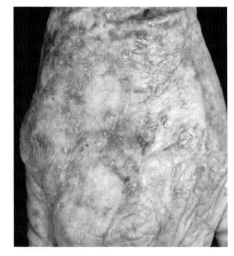

Plate 8. Actinic keratosis. These lesions are precancerous. Note the patchy redness with dry scaling skin overlying.

agents. Unfortunately, it frequently provoked allergic reactions that limited its usefulness. With the advent of the new hypoallergenic compounds, PABA has largely been replaced.

27. How do I choose the best sunscreen?

First, be sure that you're selecting a broad-spectrum sunscreen that blocks both UVA and UVB radiation. Not all products block both spectrums, so check the labels carefully. Next, consider what SPF you need. To some degree this depends upon your ability to tan. If you tan well, you may need less protection than those who burn. However, it's important to remember that a tan has an SPF of only 3 to 5. Therefore, all individuals should use sunscreen. It's recommended that you select a product with an SPF of at least 15 or 20. You should also consider your activity level. If you're active in the sun, you should select a water-resistant product. Keep in mind that all of these products eventually wash off, so you're subject to loss of protection. This is especially true in settings such as swimming or active exercise with frequent toweling off. Although the loss of protection varies from product to product and there are no general rules to apply, the longer you are active the more protection you will lose. In some cases, a product need only be effective for 90 minutes to meet the requirements for the claim that it is an "all day" sunscreen. Finally, decide between a cream- or gel-based product. If you have oily skin and are prone to develop acne, you may break out if you use a cream-based product. You may want to select a gel-based product. Conversely, if you have dry skin, a cream-based product is likely to be better for your skin.

Be sure that you're selecting a broad-spectrum sunscreen.

28. How do I maximize the benefit that a sunscreen can offer?

You can take certain steps to get the most out of your sunscreen. After you have selected the sunscreen that is best for you, you should get in the habit of using it every day. Many of us remember to put sunscreen on when we're going to the beach but neglect to use it other times. You can experience significant UV exposure on sunny days even if you're not planning to spend a long period of time in the sun. The time you spend going from the house to the car to the store can add up to extensive UV exposure. This is especially true in the areas of the country where there's a lot of sun. Also, don't be fooled by cloudy days. Approximately 85% of the sun's UV radiation will penetrate the cloud cover and reach the Earth's surface. Apply the sunscreen at least 15 minutes before you're planning to go out. Many sunscreens require a chemical reaction to occur for maximum protection, and it's important to account for this. Reapply the product every 90 to 120 minutes because most products will wash off, especially when you're doing high-energy activities such as swimming and running. This is true even for "waterproof" products. The last thing to keep in mind is that we should not use a sunscreen to extend our time in the sun, as there is concern that over time this will still increase our overall UV exposure.

Get in the habit of using sunscreen every day.

29. Do the same rules apply for my children?

In general, children's skin is more sensitive to UV-induced damage. This is especially true of very young children. Most pediatricians don't recommend using sunscreens on infants until they reach the age of 6 months. Infant skin is very thin and during this time it's best to avoid sun exposure as much as possible. Ask your pediatrician when it's appropriate to begin using a sunscreen to protect your child's skin. Otherwise the above recommendations apply especially to children. Remember that 85% of the average individual's lifetime exposure to the sun occurs before the age of 18. Additionally, recent research suggests that UV-induced damage before the ages of 12 to 15 is responsible for the development of melanoma in later years. Therefore, one of the most important things you can do is to develop good sun protection habits in your children and limit their sun exposure. To ensure the best protection possible for your child, be sure he or she wears a hat, sunglasses, and protective clothing in addition to using sunscreens regularly. Young children (ages six months to five years) usually have thinner and shorter hair, so it's necessary to protect their head, ears, and neck—areas that are frequently forgotten.

Eyes must also be protected because 2,500 cases of ocular melanoma occur every year. Wearing a wide brim hat and sunglasses that have UVA and UVB protection can do this. Even very small children can benefit from wearing sunglasses.

30. Do I need to use a sunscreen on cloudy days?

One of the most common misconceptions about sun exposure is that cloudy days provide extra protection so wearing sunscreen isn't necessary. Nothing could be further from the truth! As much as 85% of the UV rays penetrate clouds and reach the Earth's surface, causing significant sunburn damage. In fact, because of

UV-induced damage before the ages of 12 to 15 is responsible for the development of melanoma in later years.

Prevention and Protection

41

this false sense of security individuals are likely to spend more time outside, which can actually increase their risk of skin cancer.

31. I have heard that Vitamin D is made in the skin, and that it's the result of a reaction that requires UV radiation. Will using sunscreens make me deficient in this vitamin?

No! Although we do need sun exposure for good health, any additional exposure is unnecessary from a health perspective. The last step in the formation of vitamin D in the skin is the result of UV exposure. However, we make all of the vitamin D that we need in 15 minutes of sun exposure per day. Recent studies have confirmed that there is no difference in the amount of Vitamin D in individuals who use sunscreens regularly compared to those who don't.

PART FOUR

Detecting and Diagnosing Skin Cancer

How is skin cancer diagnosed?

What should I look for to determine if a mole is a melanoma?

I have a mole that I think has changed. What is my next step?

More ...

32. How is skin cancer diagnosed?

Jodie's comment:

In October of 1999, I was showing off my tattoo to a coworker when she noticed something on my shoulder. I had noticed it also, a few months earlier. I am not exactly sure how long it had been there. When looking at it, you wouldn't really think that it was once a mole. It did not look anything like a mole anymore. It was black, not tan like it used to be, and it was not smooth or oval shaped. Along with the irregular borders and dark appearance, it had begun to itch. I was very careful with it so I wouldn't make it bleed. It was under my bra strap, so I kept adjusting the strap so that it would not rub on it.

One day, I got a call from one of my coworkers telling me that another coworker had made an appointment for me to see a dermatologist. I was quite surprised. It was almost an intrusion. Not since my mom had made my doctor's appointments had anyone else done that. But I thought, okay—it was probably not a bad idea.

In Jodie's case, her coworker's action, intrusive though it might have been, probably saved her life: the mark on her skin was melanoma. As with most cancers, early detection and treatment of all skin cancers, including melanoma, is the key to treating and curing the patient. In theory, this should make melanoma one of the least dangerous cancers because changes to the skin that signify cancer are usually visible. However, this is not the case. First, if people are going to catch the signs of melanoma, they need to regularly check for skin changes. Second, they need to know what to look for so they can ask their physicians whether a change is cause for concern. Obviously, if a person isn't checking his or her skin (or going to a physician at least once a year so the physician can check), then any changes that could signify cancer will go unobserved. So the most important first step in diagnosing melanoma or other skin cancers is to check your skin for changes, and speak to your physician if you observe any. As for the second part—how you know what to look for—some of the warning signs of cancer are described in Question 33.

Check your skin for changes, and speak to your physician if you observe any.

Detecting a lesion is the first step; second comes diagnosis of the lesion as either cancerous or benign (that is, a noncancerous growth that is not cause for concern). There are some lesions that, based on their overall appearance, are easily diagnosed as cancerous or benign by your physician. However, in some instances the lesion may need to be investigated under a microscope. This is done by a procedure called a biopsy. The biopsy can be done using a variety of techniques, including Mohs' micrographic surgery as well as punch, shave, incisional, and excisional biopsies. The common denominator is that they all result in providing a piece of tissue to a physician called a **pathologist** who is responsible for making the diagnosis (see Questions 36 and 37 for more information on biopsies).

Pathologist

A physician with special training in diagnosing disease by examining tissue under the microscope.

33. What should I look for to determine if a mole is a melanoma?

There are several things to look for in a mole to determine if it should be further evaluated. The easy way to remember the important signs is to use the mnemonic ABCD, as follows:

A = asymmetry; one half of the lesion appears structurally different from the other;

B = border; the edge of the lesion is irregular in shape as if there have been "bites" taken out of it;

C = color; the color is black or shades of blue, red, maroon or several shades of brown;

D = diameter; a mole that is bigger than 6 mm in diameter (bigger than the diameter of a standard pencil eraser).

Other signs include a change in size, shape, or color, or a lesion that has become itchy or has bled. Any of the above signs or changes should prompt evaluation by your physician. Your physician will then determine if a biopsy is necessary. The only way to truly diagnose melanoma is through a biopsy that is evaluated by a pathologist.

34. I have a mole that I think has changed. What is my next step?

If you're concerned about a changing mole, the first thing to do is to seek the advice of your physician. In most cases this should be your primary care physician. Depending on their comfort level and level of training, primary care physicians may evaluate the lesion themselves or they may refer you to a dermatologist. In many cases, your physician will be able to immediately make the diagnosis and determine the appropriate treatment. In other cases, it may require a biopsy to determine the nature of the lesion. Don't manipulate the lesion in any way. In particular, don't stick the lesion with a pin or other sharp instrument. This may increase the risk of spreading the disease if the lesion is malignant.

*Don't manip-
ulate the lesion
in any way.*

When the biopsy is done, it can take anywhere from 2 to 7 days to get the diagnostic report back. This can be a stressful time for patients, but it's important to allow enough time for appropriate examination of the lesion. If a lesion is particularly unusual in its appearance, it may be sent out to a referral center for further examination. Such additional evaluation is important if the diagnosis is in question. In some cases, it may be in your best interest to ask for a second opinion. This is especially true for patients with suspected melanoma. A recent study reported that melanomas are misdiagnosed in as many as 10% of cases.

After the diagnosis is made, your physician should discuss the results with you and make any plans for additional treatment that may be necessary. Don't hesitate to ask questions if you're unsure of the plan. You have a right to be well informed about any issue pertaining to your health.

Don't hesitate to ask questions if you're unsure of the plan.

Jodie's comment:

I remember leaving the real estate office where I work and going to that appointment. I was so naïve. I had no idea what was about to happen. To this day, I regret not having someone go with me.

Everyone in the doctor's office was very nice. It seemed as though the doctor was hardly done introducing himself when he said, "That looks like melanoma." I didn't know what that was, but it didn't sound good. I became very scared. I noticed that when he would leave the room, whether it was to get the camera to take a picture of it or to get the magnifying glasses, one of his staff stayed with me as the tears were streaming down my face. I was not alone for the rest of the visit.

My doctor then proceeded to explain that he was going to take it off and send it to a pathologist to see if it was cancerous. At 27 years old, I could not believe my ears. Cancer?!

I don't remember much of the drive home except that it was hard to see through my tears. This was the scariest time of my life so far. I was waiting to hear if I had cancer.

35. I went to my physician and he told me not to worry about this lesion. It's still changing. What should I do?

It's perfectly appropriate to ask for a second opinion.

If, after an evaluation by your physician, a mole continues to be of concern to you, it's perfectly appropriate to ask for a second opinion. Sometimes, the changes in a mole may be subtle and escape early detection. In many cases, the only way to be certain of the identity of a lesion is to perform a biopsy. If you remain concerned about a mole after an evaluation by your physician, seek another opinion. History has shown that early melanomas may be missed. You're your own best advocate. Don't quit seeking help if you're dissatisfied.

36. How is a biopsy done?

Your physician decides which particular technique to use before actually doing the biopsy. The type of biopsy performed depends on several factors including the size and location of the lesion. The biopsy is done using sterile technique. That is, the area undergoing biopsy is cleaned with a medication that kills all of the bacteria that are on your skin. The surgeon's hands are also cleaned using an antibacterial soap. The surgeon then puts on sterile gloves. The biopsy area is injected with an anesthetic that deadens the nerves. This allows the procedure to be done without pain. Sometimes the area can simply be left alone to heal. However, if the lesion is large or deep, stitches may be needed to allow for complete healing and to decrease the risk of infection. When the surgery is complete, the wound is covered with an antibiotic ointment and a sterile dressing. After 1 to 2 hours the anesthetic wears off and you may feel some discomfort. If you feel discomfort, your physician will prescribe a painkiller. If the procedure was relatively minor, an over-the-counter pain medication may be suggested. More extensive procedures may require some kind of narcotic medication, such as acetaminophen plus codeine.

37. What are the different types of biopsy techniques?

There are several different approaches to performing a biopsy. The type of biopsy performed depends on a number of factors. A prerequisite of any good biopsy technique is to adequately anesthetize (numb) the site to be biopsied before starting to cut. The more common techniques are:

- *Shave:* The easiest and one of the most commonly employed of biopsy techniques is the use of the shave biopsy. In this approach, the lesion is elevated from the skin with a pair of forceps. A scalpel is used to cut the lesion away from the underlying tissue. The major problem with this approach is that some of the lesion may be left behind. Another procedure may be necessary to remove the remnant.

- *Punch:* Punch biopsies are commonly done when a lesion is small and can be contained in the specimen. Punch biopsies are also used for larger lesions that have a particular area of the lesion in question. The tool used for this technique resembles a small tube with a very sharp edge and is referred to as a punch scalpel. It comes in several different diameters to allow for different sized lesions. During the procedure, the sharp edge of the tool is twisted, cutting into the skin. Scissors are then used to remove the last portion of tissue attached to the skin

- *Incisional:* When a large lesion is on an area of the body that might require more specialized surgery (such as on the face), the surgeon may elect to do an incisional biopsy. In this technique, a scalpel removes only a portion of the lesion to obtain the questionable tissue.

- *Excisional:* When the size of the lesion is manageable, the entire lesion can be removed using a scalpel and scissors. In this procedure, the biopsied lesion is also surrounded with some portion of normal appearing tissue. The lesion and the surrounding normal tissue are sent to the pathologist.

In general, it's appropriate to submit any tissue that is removed for evaluation to the pathologist. This ensures that a diagnosis will be established. In some situations, it may be reasonable not to submit the tissue for evaluation. However, you must make sure that you understand whether or not your specimen will go to the pathologist. If your specimen isn't going to a pathologist, ask why.

If your specimen isn't going to a pathologist, ask why.

38. I have been scheduled for Mohs' surgery. What does this mean?

When surgeons remove suspected malignant lesions, they also usually remove some of the surrounding normal tissue. This is done to make sure that no malignant cells are left behind. When there's no tumor at the edge of the tissue, the tissue is said to have clear margins. If the surgical site is on the back, for instance, there is usually adequate tissue to accomplish this and still close the wound without using a **skin graft** or other more involved surgical techniques. In some situations, however, there's a need to limit the amount of tissue that's removed during surgery. For example, if the lesion is on the face, taking too much normal tissue may cause disfigurement. To deal with this situation, Dr. Mohs developed a technique wherein the tissue is immediately examined under the microscope to make sure the margins are clear. During the surgery, a narrow margin of what appears to be normal skin is defined. The surgeon then cuts along this margin. The tissue that is removed is evaluated under the microscope and if the margins are clear the wound is closed. However, if the margin is positive (contains malignant cells), the surgeon removes more tissue. This process is repeated until all margins are clear. Mohs' surgery usually requires patients to be at the facility for several hours. The approach is commonly used to remove basal and squamous cell cancers. Its role in treating patients with malignant melanoma is more controversial.

Skin graft

A procedure wherein a piece of skin is removed from what is referred to as a donor site and transferred to an area where a surgical procedure has removed enough tissue to prevent it from being closed without a significant defect. The donor site heals but a scar is left behind.

Detecting and Diagnosing Skin Cancer

PART FIVE

What Does It Mean to Have Melanoma?

Are there different kinds of melanoma?

Is one type of melanoma more dangerous than another?

More ...

39. Are there different kinds of melanoma?

Most melanomas begin in the skin and are referred to as cutaneous melanomas. However, melanoma can begin in the eye (ocular melanoma) as well as in places such as the mouth, rectum, and vagina. The latter are referred to as mucosal melanomas.

Ocular melanomas occur in approximately 2,500 individuals each year. One of the most common symptoms is loss of vision in all or part of an eye. These melanomas commonly spread to the liver if they aren't diagnosed early. Most often, such melanomas are treated initially by ophthalmologists (eye specialists). In rare situations, patients will be diagnosed with both ocular and cutaneous forms of melanoma. If you're diagnosed with a skin melanoma, it's a good idea to have an eye examination to determine if there are any concerns regarding the eyes.

Mucosal melanomas can be difficult to diagnose and frequently aren't found until they have spread. The symptoms may differ depending on where the mucosal melanomas start, which is why this form of melanoma is particularly dangerous.

Cutaneous melanomas are further classified on the basis of their appearance under the microscope:

- *Superficial spreading:* Superficial spreading melanoma (Plate 5) is the most common form of this disease, representing approximately 40% of all cutaneous melanomas. These lesions tend to grow along the skin for a long period of time before they begin to invade deeper into the skin. They are typically irregular in shape and several shades of brown. They may have other colors such as black, blue, or red.

- *Nodular:* Nodular melanomas (Plate 6) are typically dome-shaped lesions that are black in color and elevated above the level of the skin. They tend to change size quickly and may be associated with smaller lesions located close by. These smaller lesions are called satellite lesions and represent local spread.

- *Lentigo malignant:* Lentigo malignant melanomas are most common in the elderly population. These lesions are typically flat and spread widely along the surface of the skin. Lentigo malignant melanomas often begin as non-malignant lesions (lentigo maligna) that are found on the face or other sun exposed area.

- *Acral lentigenous:* Acral lentigenous melanoma (Plate 7) is usually found underneath the fingernails and toenails or on the palms of the hands or soles of the feet. This is the form of melanoma that's most common in individuals who have naturally pigmented skin. It's very important to pay attention to dark lesions under the nails especially if there is no prior history of trauma to the area. A dark area under a nail that is related to trauma usually grows out with the nail. If a lesion doesn't grow out, it should be considered for biopsy.

- *Desmoplastic/Neurotropic:* Desmoplastic or neurotropic melanomas are unusual variants that have a propensity to provoke the development of fibrous tissue in addition to seeking out nerves in the skin to grow and travel alongside of them. These variants have a somewhat higher risk for coming back in the same area. They also show themselves as small nodules in the skin.

- *Amelanotic melanoma:* Amelanotic melanomas are melanomas that don't make pigment. They're frequently pink or flesh-colored. Unfortunately, because they don't make pigment, amelanotic melanomas are commonly misdiagnosed as pimples or other non-malignant lesions.

40. Why is malignant melanoma so dangerous?

Of the three most common skin cancers, malignant melanoma represents the only truly life-threatening form. As mentioned earlier, this disease stems from melanocytes, the cells that produce melanin in response to UV radiation. Initially, melanoma spreads along the surface of the skin. This is called the horizontal growth phase. This growth phase can last months to years, depending on the type of melanoma involved. The melanoma subsequently begins to invade the skin in a process called the vertical growth phase. During this phase of growth, the melanoma cells gain access to blood and lymphatic vessels, allowing the cells to travel to other parts of the body. After the melanoma cells spread, the chance for cure decreases significantly. The melanoma cells invade normal tissues and destroy them by infiltrating and replacing the normal cells. In contrast, the great majority of basal and squamous cancer cells don't have this ability to spread and therefore only invade locally. This distinction accounts for the substantial difference in prognosis between the different types of skin cancers.

41. Is one type of melanoma more dangerous than another?

Historically, many physicians have felt that nodular melanomas carry a worse prognosis than any of the other types of melanoma. However, stage for stage, the risk is equal for equivalent lesions. All other things being equal, a 1 millimeter (mm) thick nodular melanoma carries the same prognosis as a 1 mm super-ficial spreading melanoma. What's different about nodular melanoma is how it grows. We mentioned above the horizontal and vertical growth phases of melanoma. During the horizontal growth phase, the melanoma is growing along the skin and hasn't yet invaded it; there's no risk of the melanoma spreading to other parts of the body. When the melanoma enters the vertical growth phase it has learned to invade and it can spread to other organs. Superficial spreading melanomas typically spend many months to years in the horizontal growth phase; thus they are unable to spread. In con-trast, nodular melanomas quickly leave the horizontal growth phase (sometimes after only several months) and enter the vertical growth phase. Therefore, nodular melanomas can metastasize to other parts of the body much earlier than the other types of melanoma.

42. Are my family members at risk because I have been diagnosed with melanoma?

The sun causes melanoma, so there's no chance that a family member can "catch" this disease. Additionally, melanoma can't be passed through close or sexual con-tact. However, there are situations in which family members carry a similar risk of melanoma as a result of shared genes. The most well-defined inherited melanoma syndrome is the dysplastic nevus syndrome, also known as familial atypical mole melanoma syn-drome. Families with this syndrome develop abnormal or dysplastic moles that have a high predisposition to malignant degeneration.

Affected family members have a genetic mutation found on chromosome 9 in the *p16* gene. Parents with an abnormality of this gene pass it on to their children in high frequency. The normal *p16* gene is referred to as a tumor suppressor gene. When they function normally, tumor suppressor genes act to prevent the development of cancer. Their presence and activity are necessary to prevent damaged cells from replicating and ultimately becoming malignant. In this case, the product of the *p16* gene is a protein that prevents cells with damaged DNA from making new cells. If the protein is missing, cells with damaged DNA can replicate, thereby increasing the risk of malignant degeneration. Not all families with this syndrome have the same abnormality of the *p16* gene; therefore, there must be additional genes that can result in a similar predisposition to the development of the same syndrome. All immediate family members of a newly diagnosed melanoma patient should undergo a complete head-to-toe skin screening to determine if they are at risk for developing a melanoma. This is recommended regardless of whether or not an abnormal mole pattern exists in the family.

43. I developed a melanoma during my pregnancy. Did my pregnancy cause my melanoma? Could I give it to my baby?

There's no evidence to suggest that pregnancy causes melanoma to form. Additionally, there's no evidence to support that patients who develop melanoma during pregnancy have a worse outcome compared to women who develop melanoma unrelated to pregnancy. Despite a lack of clear evidence to the contrary, many physicians believe that there is a small subpopulation of women whose melanoma grows more rapidly during pregnancy. Melanocytes contain hormone receptors and are stimulated to produce more pigment during pregnancy. Melanoma cells also contain hormone receptors. The theory is that melanoma cells may be stimulated to proliferate more rapidly in response to the marked elevation of hormones during pregnancy. Physicians who take care of many melanoma patients can point to several cases that support this concept.

Many physicians will recommend that a young woman who has been recently diagnosed with a melanoma wait at least 2 years before becoming pregnant again. This is recommended in an attempt to decrease the risk that the melanoma would return during pregnancy. In general, approximately 80% of those individuals who suffer the recurrence of their melanoma will do so within 2 years of their initial diagnosis. By waiting 2 years to become pregnant again, the majority of patients can avoid this situation.

Malignant melanoma is an uncommon tumor during pregnancy, accounting for only 8% of malignancies in pregnant women. Even fewer patients have metastatic melanoma during pregnancy. Melanoma is commonly found in the placenta, but it rarely crosses this organ to reach the unborn child.

44. How do you cope when diagnosed with malignant melanoma?

Jodie's comment:

I was able to cope with this diagnosis through a strong support system along with a group of wonderful and caring doctors. My family was great. I cannot count the times mom and I have cried together. That was not something that we had ever done before and was absolutely necessary from my perspective. It was always a healing cry. My boyfriend was there for me, and his family was as well. It made such a tremendous difference. I knew I could make it through this when the people around me were constantly telling me I could.

Everyone's methods of coping are different, and there's no one strategy that will work for all people diagnosed with this disease. But as Jodie points out above, the key to coping successfully with any serious illness is *don't try to do it alone.* Melanoma is not a disease to be "toughed out." If you find yourself feeling anxious, sad, or depressed, don't be ashamed or think you must suffer through these feelings alone—they're entirely normal reactions to a very difficult situation, and with proper assistance they can be alleviated. Ask your doctor or nurse to refer you to a counselor (hospitals often have a social worker specializing in helping cancer patients), or talk to a minister or mental health professional. Your loved ones can be of great help to you—if you let them. Even if you feel unable to confide in a family member or counselor, there are resources available to help you: organizations such as the American Cancer Society, the National Coalition for Cancer Survivorship, and the American Melanoma Foundation, among others, provide many kinds of resources for melanoma patients, from Internet chat rooms to educational materials to practical advice on what to do about your illness. The Appendix to this book lists a variety of resources that can be very helpful. Use them!

PART SIX

Treatment of Malignant Melanoma

I've been diagnosed with malignant melanoma. What do I do now?

What is the role of the pathologist in my care?

What are the prognostic factors that I need to know about?

More ...

45. I've been diagnosed with malignant melanoma. What do I do now?

Jodie's comment:

When the doctor's office called me two days after my biopsy, I made a regular "just need to see you" appointment. But before I got off the phone with her, I put her on the spot. I said, "Please tell me if it was positive. I need to know." She then told me, in such a nice way, that yes, it did come back cancerous. At that point, I had to call my mom, who was at work waiting for my call. I waited for two hours before I could talk to her. I couldn't stop crying. I kept myself composed through the conversation with the receptionist, but as soon as I heard my mother's voice, I once again burst into tears. I said, "Mom, my tests were positive, but I'm all right." I honestly can't remember what she said. I was kind of in a fog.

You will need to move forward quickly to start treatment.

First, take a deep breath and recognize that most patients with melanoma are cured. Like Jodie, you may be frightened, but once the initial shock is over you will need to move forward quickly to start treatment; melanoma is not a disease that permits delay. As soon as possible, make a plan with your physician as to what your next steps should be. In general, your physician will begin to collect information regarding the pathologist's interpretation of your melanoma. These are referred to as prognostic factors. Basically, they represent specific findings that help your physician determine how serious your particular melanoma is. Next, you may be referred to a surgeon for what's called a wide re-excision (see Question 49). In addition, it will be determined whether you'll need to undergo a **sentinel lymph node biopsy**. When the prognostic factors and sentinel lymph node biopsy results are available,

Sentinel lymph node biopsy

A procedure designed to identify the most likely lymph node to contain metastatic melanoma cells.

the risk of the cancer spreading to other parts of your body will be determined. If that risk is high, you'll be offered what's called **adjuvant therapy** or preventive therapy to decrease the risk that the disease will return. If the risk of the cancer spreading is small, you'll be entered into a follow-up program that will monitor you over time.

46. What is the role of the pathologist in my care?

After your physician has performed the biopsy, the tissue is sent for examination under a microscope by a physician called a pathologist, who has special training to diagnose disease by examining tissues. The pathologist will make the diagnosis and should also provide your physician with your prognostic factors. These factors can help determine if you need additional treatment beyond the surgery to remove the melanoma on your skin.

47. What are the prognostic factors that I need to know about?

The pathologist will first determine what type of melanoma you have. Next, the invasive nature of the lesion will be documented either as a **Clark's level** or as a **Breslow's thickness** (see Question 48). The pathologist should discuss other issues that are important to your physician including determining the **mitotic index**, the presence or absence of **tumor infiltrating lymphocytes (TILs)**, and whether or not there

Adjuvant therapy

Clinical setting in which all visible evidence of disease has been removed, but the patient remains at high risk for the disease to return elsewhere in the body.

Clark's level

A measurement of tumor penetration into skin layers.

Breslow's thickness

A staging system that relies on the thickness of the tumor.

Mitotic Index

A count of the number of mitotic figures that can be found in a square millimeter of the primary pathologic tissue.

Tumor infiltrating lymphocytes (TILs)

Lymphocytes that invade into melanoma.

is regression or ulceration. This is the first step in what is called the staging process. When your physician talks with you about your melanoma, the stage of your disease will be discussed. This is another way of discussing how far the tumor has spread from the original or primary site. As discussed earlier, the danger of melanoma is that it will metastasize from the primary site to different areas of the body. Your physician will attempt to determine how far your tumor has spread. This will determine the stage of your disease.

There are basically two staging systems that are used in melanoma. The first system has been designed to provide risk assessment information based on the primary tumor itself. Important issues here include the Clark's level or Breslow's thickness of invasion, the location of the tumor, the gender of the patient, the mitotic index, and whether or not there are TILs or evidence of regression and ulceration. The second staging system has been designed to provide information about risk assessment as it relates to the entire body. This system is referred to as the TNM system. "T" stands for tumor, "N" stands for lymph nodes, and "M" stands for metastases to other sites of the body. This system is quite involved. A brief overview of cancer staging follows.

- Stages I and II refer to disease that's limited to the primary site in the skin only.
- Stage III represents disease that has spread beyond the primary site to involve local skin or lymph nodes that are close by the primary site.
- Stage IV represents disease that has spread to other organs of the body.

The higher the cancer stage, the greater the risk that the disease spread before it was removed, and the greater the risk of death from the disease.

48. What is the difference between Clark's level and Breslow's thickness?

The Clark's level uses the skin's natural anatomy to determine how deep the tumor has penetrated. The Clark's levels for skin are described below.

- Level 1 lesions grow along what's called the dermal/epidermal junction. They don't have metastatic potential because they haven't invaded skin. Level I lesions can't spread because there are no blood or lymphatic vessels in the epidermis, which means that the lesions have no means of transport out of the area in which they originated except to grow directly into surrounding tissue. Level I lesions pose no risk to life.
- Level II lesions have broken through the dermal/epidermal junction to invade the most superficial layer of the dermis, called the papillary layer, but they don't invade it completely. Level II lesions are the first to encounter blood or lymphatic vessels and represent the first level of invasion that may be associated with spread. However, these lesions usually carry a low risk for metastasis.
- Level III lesions invade deeper into the skin and extend to the border of the papillary and reticular layers of the dermis. The risk of metastatic spread begins to increase with lesions that invade this deep.
- Level IV lesions invade directly into the reticular layer of the dermis but don't reach the subcutaneous

tissue. The risk for spread of this lesion is higher than that for level III lesions. Other prognostic factors, such as **mitotic figures** and tumor infiltrating lymphocytes, are important to consider with this lesion in order to determine the risk of metastasis.

- Level V lesions have invaded directly into the sub-cutaneous tissue and generally carry a high risk of metastasis.

The above cutaneous staging system has been used for many years and provides valuable information to physicians. However, determining a level III melanoma from a level IV melanoma is sometimes very difficult. Distinguishing between the two levels is important because the prognosis is different for each. Dr. Breslow suggested a different staging system that's based strictly on the measured thickness of the melanoma and doesn't require determining the different layers of the skin. A measurement device is now incorporated into the microscope's eyepiece. This measurement device allows the pathologist to directly measure the thickness of the melanoma. The depth is measured and then reported to your physician. The report includes the actual depth of invasion as well as a classification of the invasion according to the T staging system. The T stages are defined as follows:

- T0: A melanoma that hasn't invaded; also called a melanoma in situ
- T1: A tumor that is 1 mm thick or less
- T2: A tumor that is more than 1 mm (but no more than 2 mm) thick
- T3: A tumor that is more than 2 mm (but no more than 4 mm) thick

Mitotic figure

A cell that has condensed DNA in the form of a chromosome that is visible under the microscope.

- T4: A tumor that is more than 4 mm thick

Your physician then uses the information obtained in the biopsy to plan additional wide re-excision surgery. In most cases, the Breslow's thickness is more predictive of survival. When your physician receives the pathology report, both the Clark's level and the Breslow's thickness are provided. Your physician will rely more heavily on the Breslow's thickness to predict your survival and to plan future treatment.

49. They tell me that I must have another surgical procedure called a wide re-excision. Why didn't they take enough out the first time?

The standard surgical approach for treating malignant melanoma is to remove the lesion in two steps. This approach is taken even when the diagnosis of melanoma is suspected before the biopsy is performed. The reason for this approach is that information obtained from the original biopsy is used in the second procedure called the wide re-excision. Melanoma has a tendency to recur at the primary site (often called local recurrence) after it acquires the ability to invade deeper into the skin. Some melanoma cells migrate, but still remain relatively close to the primary site. The deeper the invasion, the higher the risk of a local recurrence. If the migrated melanoma cells aren't removed along with the primary lesion, a local tumor recurrence will occur. Patients who suffer local recurrence are at higher risk to develop further sites of metastases and ultimately die of metastatic disease. Therefore, every effort is made to remove all of the melanoma at the onset of treatment to allow for the earliest initiation of adjuvant therapy if appropriate.

When melanoma is suspected, the surgeon plans to remove the entire visible lesion in surgery. The removed tissue is then sent to the pathologist, who determines how deep the melanoma has invaded into the skin. The depth of invasion is then used to determine how much more normal tissue must be removed in an attempt to remove any cells that may have separated from the primary site but still remain in the local vicinity. Table 3 shows guidelines that help determine how much tissue is removed.

Note that these are only guidelines; they are not strict rules for wide re-excision. Depending on the clinical situation, more or less tissue may be removed. For example, a melanoma on the face (especially one close to the eye or nose) may require a wide re-excision that would cause significant cosmetic damage or be technically impossible. In this situation, less of the normal tissue is removed. In other cases, more tissue may need to be removed in order to obtain a good cosmetic closure of the wound. It's important that you discuss these issues with your physician as well as understand the rationale for any decisions regarding compromise of the recommended margin.

Table 3.   Guidelines for wide re-excision

Depth of invasion	Margin of wide re-excision
Melanoma in situ	0.5 cm
≤ 2 mm	1.0 cm
≥ 2.1 mm	2.0 cm

50. How do I select a surgeon?

Jodie's comment:

When the doctor talked with me that first day, he told me that there was a plan for my next step. That helped me to cope with the devastation. Because the tests were positive, the next step would be to meet my surgeon.

The surgeon introduced himself to my mom and my boyfriend, then walked over to me. I was sitting in a chair a few steps away. He started to talk to me, but to my surprise I started to cry again. He said, "What's wrong?" I remember thinking, "What the hell do you think is wrong with me?!" but what I was able to spit out was, "I'm so scared!" He quickly pulled up a chair and held my hand and said, "I know you are, but we can fix you." That was the best thing anyone could have said to me at that time.

Depending on the location of the lesion and the extent of the surgery required, your wide re-excision may be done by either a dermatologist or a surgeon. Most dermatologists will not perform large wide re-excisions or sentinel lymph node dissections. In such situations you will likely be referred to a surgeon. Many times, this individual will be a surgeon who operates on patients with a variety of illnesses. In recent years, there has been rapid growth of surgical oncology as a subspecialty. Surgical oncologists (or oncologic surgeons) have trained at major cancer centers and focus their practice on operating on patients with cancer. Whether you as the patient should seek out a surgeon who specializes in cancer surgery is a commonly asked question. The fact of the matter is that most cancer surgery in the United States today is performed by well-trained individuals who have the technical expertise to perform the required procedure. Given this fact, it's important to rely on the advice of your primary care physician to help you select the right individual. There are times, however, when the clinical situation is such that it requires the advice and technical expertise of a surgeon who specializes in cancer surgery. Again, your primary care physician should help you find a physician with the skill to perform the procedure necessary to give you the best chance for survival.

51. I have been told that I need a sentinel lymph node biopsy. What is this for?

Jodie's comment:

After I met with my surgeon, I was told that the next step was to take some lymph nodes out to see if the cancer had spread. It's called a sentinel lymph node biopsy. If that test came back positive, I would have all of the nodes in my right armpit removed—a complete right axillary lymphadenectomy.

Two weeks after being diagnosed, I went in for my first ever surgery. My surgeon took out seven nodes. I remember seeing the disappointment on his face when he had to tell me that the test came back positive. Two of the seven nodes were positive for cancer.

As melanoma cells invade into the skin, they encounter blood and lymphatic vessels. Upon entering the vessel, the cells are carried throughout the body and can spread to other sites and organs. One of the most common sites of spread is to lymph nodes, especially lymph nodes that are close to where the melanoma started.

It turns out that within any lymph node group, there are one or two lymph nodes that are the first to be encountered by a melanoma cell that is metastasizing from the primary site. This lymph node is referred to as the **sentinel lymph node**. Recent studies have shown that by examining this lymph node under the microscope, important information is obtained that can help with decisions regarding the potential need for additional treatment. In the majority of cases, only one lymph node is found. In some cases, however, two or three sentincl lymph nodes might be identified and sent for evaluation.

In general, the surgeon schedules the sentinel lymph node biopsy to be done at the same time as the wide re-excision. This is due to the fact that the path of the lymph fluid flow is disrupted by the wide re-excision procedure. Therefore, the two procedures are done at the same time, with the sentinel lymph node biopsy completed first.

The lymph node is then sent to the pathologist, who examines the tissue to determine if there are any melanoma cells in it. If no melanoma cells are in the lymph node, then there's a less than 5% chance that melanoma will ever be found in that lymph node group. This also suggests that there's less of a chance that the melanoma has spread anywhere else in the body.

A sentinel lymph node procedure consists of the following steps:

- *Lymphoscintigraphy:* Before beginning the procedure, the surgeon must know which lymph nodes

Sentinel lymph node

The lymph node in a lymph node basin that is the first lymph node encountered by a tumor cell entering that basin.

Treatment of Malignant Melanoma

drain the primary melanoma site. If the lesion was on your arm or hand, the lymph node area is usually located in the armpit (axilla). If the melanoma involved your leg or foot, the lymph node area would be the groin. However, if the melanoma is on the torso or the head and neck region then the drainage is more ambiguous. A melanoma on your upper chest may metastasize to either axilla or into the neck area. The lymphoscintigraphy helps to define where the melanoma is most likely to have metastasized. The procedure involves injecting a radioactive material into the skin surrounding the primary melanoma site. The radioactive material follows the same path that the melanoma cell would travel and winds up in the draining lymph node basins. You're then placed under a scanner that is sensitive to the radioactive substance. Pictures are taken that will show which lymph nodes are most likely to be involved with metastatic disease. In most cases only one site is identified; however, it's common for more than one site to be involved. This procedure is done within a few days of the actual sentinel lymph node biopsy.

- *Sentinel lymph node biopsy:* The actual biopsy is typically done at the same time as the wide re-excision. Before removing the primary melanoma, the site is again injected with both a radioactive substance as well as a blue dye. The surgeon uses a hand held Geiger counter to detect the most radioactive site in the lymph node basin and makes a small incision at that site. The surgeon then identifies lymphatic channels carrying the blue dye and follows them until a lymph node is found. The Geiger counter is used to check for radioactivity in the lymph node.

Assuming it's positive, the lymph node is removed and sent to the pathologist. If no other radioactive lymph nodes are found, the procedure is completed and the wound is closed. In some cases, a second or even a third radioactive lymph node is removed and sent to the pathologist for examination.

- *Pathologic examination:* Key to the success of this procedure is adequate examination of the sentinel lymph node by the pathologist. The lymph node specimen is cut into many small sections, which are then examined under the microscope for evidence of melanoma cells. The results are sent to your surgeon.

Jodie's comment:

Two weeks after the sentinel lymph node biopsy, I had 30 lymph nodes removed. What an experience that was! I had a drain to empty every few hours for a week, and I couldn't move my arm without pain (so I didn't!). I had to work on moving and lifting my arm. It took a few weeks before I could even brush my hair again. I did finger climbing exercises up the wall until I could reach straight up. I needed help getting dressed. I had to brush my teeth with my left hand.

If evidence of melanoma is found, your surgeon may recommend that you have further surgery to remove the remaining lymph nodes in the area. It's not yet clear that there is any benefit in doing this additional procedure; however, many surgeons prefer to go back and remove any remaining lymph nodes in an attempt to improve the patient's chance for survival.

Treatment of Malignant Melanoma

52. My surgeon has recommended an elective lymph node dissection. What is this procedure? Is it important in my care?

An elective lymph node dissection refers to a surgical procedure during which all identifiable lymph nodes in the draining lymph node basin are removed. This is done without any clear evidence that there is metastatic melanoma in the area. The draining lymph node basin is usually a lymph node area to which the melanoma cells from a particular melanoma would normally spread. For instance, a melanoma on your left arm is most likely to spread to the lymph nodes under your left arm if the melanoma cells enter the lymph system. It's critically important to understand that there is no reason that the melanoma cells have to spread via the lymph system. They may simply enter blood vessels and skip the lymph nodes in this area.

Elective lymph node dissection is performed in a manner similar to the sentinel lymph node biopsy described above. A lymphoscintigraphy may be necessary before surgery. The major difference is that during an elective lymph node procedure, the surgeon attempts to remove all lymph nodes in the area. This may add significantly to the morbidity (complications) of the procedure.

This approach is based partly on an outdated notion that melanoma cells must spread through the lymph nodes before they go elsewhere in the body, and the notion that removing these lymph nodes can cure patients. Current evidence has demonstrated that this approach offers no survival advantage over simply removing the lymph node if a tumor develops in the area. Many patients who have undergone elective lymph node dissection would never have developed melanoma in these lymph nodes, and have been subjected to an unnecessary surgical procedure. Although most patients do well postoperatively, this procedure can be associated with significant postoperative problems including infection, wound breakdown, and (in some cases) a chronically swollen extremity. Given the information available today, there is no good reason for the performance of an elective lymph node procedure.

53. My surgeon has sent me to a medical oncologist. What is this physician's role?

Jodie's comment:

*After the lymphadenectomy, I thought everything was fine. Then it was explained to me that I would need to meet my **next** doctor. I understood that I might need chemotherapy. The day my mom, my boyfriend, and I were in the office with my medical oncologist, I was like a sponge—ready to absorb the information I was about to receive.*

I liked my doctor, Dr. McClay, right away. It didn't hurt that his wife worked alongside him. They were in the room with us for what felt like two hours or so. He explained how my "tumor" grew in my body and told me that because it had gone into my lymph nodes, I was in the "high risk" zone, at high risk for the cancer to return.

After the dermatologist or surgeon has completed the surgical portion of your treatment, you may be sent to a medical oncologist for a recommendation as to whether or not you need to consider additional therapy. A medical oncologist is a physician who has specialized in the care of cancer patients. The oncologist will help to determine the risk that your melanoma has spread to other parts of the body before it was diagnosed and removed. If the risk is high, the medical oncologist will help you to determine the best treatment and will likely be responsible for administration of the treatment. Medical oncologists usually treat patients with chemotherapy, immunotherapy, or both for a defined period of time after surgery has been completed. In many cases, the medical oncologist becomes the physician who provides the majority of your care concerning your cancer treatment. Consider your medical oncologist as your primary care physician for your cancer care.

54. How do I select an oncologist?

In most cases, either your primary care physician or your surgeon will refer you to an oncologist in whom they have confidence. Your first meeting with your oncologist is a time to obtain as much information as possible about your disease as well as your new physician. It's critically important for you to feel comfortable and trust your physician. This relationship requires effort on the part of both the physician and the patient. There should be open communication and honesty in order to make sure that you as the patient feel that you can ask any question and receive correct and up-to-date answers.

It's critically important for you to feel comfortable and trust your physician.

In most cases, you should seek out a physician who is a board certified medical oncologist. A medical oncologist is a physician who has completed training in internal medicine and then received subspecialty training in the treatment of patients with cancer. Board certification means that the physician has completed subspecialty training and subsequently passed a certification examination. Sometimes older physicians have specialized in the treatment of cancer patients before formal training was available. These individuals have devoted their life to treating patients with this disease and are more than qualified to do so. The key point is to make sure that a physician with the expertise you will need to get you through this most difficult time is caring for you.

When you're discussing treatment options, it's important to understand that there are several situations in which standard therapy (treatment that is accepted and applied similarly across the country) is offered. However, in other situations the treatment you're offered may depend on the treatment philosophy of your physician. This is where it's important for you to understand exactly what your physician's treatment philosophy is and how closely it fits with yours. For example, many patients want to take an aggressive approach to their treatment from the time that the diagnosis is made. These individuals are frequently willing to tolerate significant toxicity from treatment if there is even a small chance of benefit. Other patients are more interested in their quality of life. These individuals are only willing to undergo rigorous treatment if there is a very good chance for an excellent outcome. In order for you to get the most out of the relationship, you and your physician must be on the same page in regard to the treatment approaches you prefer.

55. What questions should I ask my oncologist?

Jodie's comment:

Young women like me—a group that's at high risk for melanoma—might want to ask about the future in regard to pregnancy. Are there any foreseeable problems with fertility, such as damage to your eggs? And all people with melanoma need to ask some of the following questions: Are there any long-term effects from the treatment you chose? Are there any more options for treatments? How safe would it be if I chose to not do any treatment at all? In regards to choosing a treatment: When will the treatment(s) end? Will I lose my hair? Will I be sick? Will I be able to function normally? Will this affect my emotional behavior? How long will it take to get back to normal after treatment is over? When in treatment, should I try to not get a cold? Would that affect the treatment— maybe make it worse? What should I eat? What shouldn't I eat? Are herbal supplements or vitamins hazardous when mixed with treatment? How important is potassium during treatment?

You should come away from your first meeting with your oncologist with specific information that is important in helping you make decisions regarding your prognosis. The minimum information should include:

- How deep did the tumor invade into the skin?
- Did it reach the lymph nodes?
- What is the risk that the melanoma has spread to internal organs?
- What additional treatment is needed?

- Do you need specialized studies such as **positron-emission tomography (PET)** and or **computerized tomographic (CT) scans**? How often?
- What is the schedule for your follow-up care?
- What is your prognosis?

56. How often should I see my physician after my surgery?

Your follow-up after surgery will depend on the risk of recurrence that's been identified by the prognostic factors of the primary lesion and the results of the sentinel lymph node biopsy. If the risk that the melanoma metastasized before lesion removal is low, then you're considered a low-risk patient and require less aggressive follow-up. Keep in mind that patients who have developed melanoma have a 3% to 5% chance of developing a second primary melanoma (that is, a brand new lesion, not recurrence of the first one). Therefore, these patients need to remain in a screening program. Patients usually go for a complete head to toe skin examination as well as a complete history and a physical at least every 6 months. In some cases, it may be necessary to have more frequent evaluations as appropriate.

If the risk of spread is modest, patients are likely to have a complete examination every 3 to 4 months. If there any symptoms that suggest recurrence of the melanoma, appropriate studies such as CT or PET scans are performed.

High-risk patients are generally evaluated with a complete history and physical and skin examination every

Positron-emission tomography (PET) Scan

A test that uses a small amount of radioactive glucose to identify areas in the body that contain tumor cells. This test doesn't use X-rays.

Computerized tomographic (CT) scans

A specialized x-ray procedure that uses successive x-rays reproduced by computer to look for tumors.

Patients who have developed melanoma have a 3% to 5% chance of developing a second primary melanoma.

2 months. Additionally, CT and PET scans are performed every 4 months for the first 2 years after diagnosis. If the 2 years have passed without recurrence, visits are decreased to every 3 to 4 months and CT and PET scans are performed twice per year. In general, 85% of patients with melanoma who develop metastatic disease will do so within 2 years of their initial diagnosis. Therefore, the 2-year evaluation is very important. In some patients, but not all, the risk of metastases decreases significantly after 2 years, therefore the frequency of such testing can be decreased at that time. This, however, is a clinical decision that is made between you and your physician. There may be factors that suggest that your risk of metastases remains high even if 2 years have passed without complications.

57. My doctor has told me that I need adjuvant therapy. What does this mean?

Jodie's comment:

I now had to make a major decision. I had a few options to choose from. One was to do nothing. It's called watching and waiting—waiting for it to come back. Another was to have adjuvant therapy to boost my own immune system. Honestly, both of those scared the hell out of me. I decided that what sounded the best to me was to teach my cells to fight off the cancer cells—that is, if the cancer were to come back. I decided to join Dr. McClay's clinical trials of adjuvant therapy.

By using information that is obtained from the pathologist after examination of the tissue removed from the primary site as well as the sentinel lymph node biopsy, the risk that your melanoma has spread before it was removed can be estimated. In addition to the biopsy you may be asked to undergo specialized testing such as CT and PET scans. These highly specialized tests can find very small tumors that may have spread from the primary site located in internal organs. However, tumors that are less than 1 cm in size may be missed, even with this sophisticated testing.

All of the information obtained through testing is used to determine the risk that your tumor has spread and the likelihood that it will return at some other site. If that risk is high, you and your physician may consider employing adjuvant or preventive treatment to decrease the risk that the melanoma will return. Because the spread of melanoma is frequently associated with the ultimate death of the patient, the decision to use adjuvant therapy is an important one that must be made with as much information as is available.

Adjuvant therapy has been used to successfully treat patients with a variety of cancers, such as breast and colon cancer. In this setting, treatment is given when there is no clear evidence of a tumor. However, it is highly likely that microscopic disease exists somewhere else in the body. For patients with both types of cancer, adjuvant therapy has been shown to decrease the risk of return of the disease and improves the survival of the patients treated.

Until recently, there has not been effective adjuvant therapy for patients with melanoma. Several studies have suggested that 12 months of treatment with high-dose interferon produces a modest survival benefit (see Question 58). All physicians do not accept this; therefore, it's important to have a frank and open discussion with your physician before entering into treatment. As there are new treatments under development, your physician may suggest that you consider entering a clinical trial (see Part 7).

58. My oncologist recommended that I take interferon. What is this medicine, and what are its side effects?

Jodie's comment:

I remember my mom saying, "Take a deep breath, Jodie, and get ready for this one." Even with all the papers you have to sign that explain what you will be going through, you still really have no idea what to expect. The fear of the unknown can really kick your butt—if you let it! My treatment consisted of high doses of tamoxifen along with a stay in the hospital to receive my chemo, two days to recover from that, and then on day five I started my shots of interferon and interleukin, which were for my immune system. I'm glad I had a few days between the chemo and the shots because the shots had a lot more side effects than the chemo. They say it has "flu-like" symptoms. What a joke!! This is definitely like no flu you have ever had before! Although the symptoms might sound familiar, it feels different from the flu.

Interferon is one of the older forms of immunotherapy. It has been used for more than 20 years. In adjuvant treatment, interferon is usually administered in very high doses and should be given only by physicians with experience using this medicine. During the first month of treatment, the interferon is administered as an intravenous injection daily for five days a week. The injection is usually administered in your physician's office. After the first month, the dose is cut in half and given as an injection under the skin, three times per week for the next 48 weeks. Overall, the adjuvant therapy takes one year to complete. After the initial inter-feron injections are administered by the physician, many patients either self-inject the medication or a family member is taught how to do the injections.

Most of the side effects of interferon are referred to as "flu-like" symptoms. Thus, fevers, chills, muscle and joint aches, as well as loss of appetite nausea and vom-iting, are common. It's critically important during this time that you keep in close communication with your physician's office so that they can be of maximum assistance to you. There are many steps that can be taken to prevent (or at least lessen) the above side effects. If the side effects are problematic then the dose of the interferon is usually decreased. In some cases, patients are unable to tolerate the treatment even when the dose has been decreased, and the interferon is stopped.

As mentioned above, interferon therapy is scheduled to continue for a total of 12 months. At the end of the treatment you'll enter a follow-up program in which you'll be monitored on a regular basis to determine the success of the treatment.

59. My oncologist was talking about disease-free survival and overall survival. What is the difference?

When you talk about survival with your oncologist, it's important to make the distinction between disease-free survival and overall survival. These are two factors that your oncologist uses to determine whether or not a particular treatment will be useful in treating patients. Both begin at the time the patient is first diagnosed but have different end points. Disease-free survival begins when the patient is first diagnosed and ends when the patient's tumor returns. Overall survival begins when the patient is diagnosed and ends with the patient's death. For example, if a patient's tumor returns 18 months after they're diagnosed with cancer and he or she ultimately dies of the disease 36 months after diagnosis, the disease-free survival is 18 months and the overall survival is 36 months. Obviously, most patients are interested in overall survival because they are interested in prolonging their life. However, both forms of survival are measured in most clinical trials, so you must be certain that you understand which type of survival your physician is talking about.

60. Where does melanoma usually spread?

Once the melanoma cells have acquired the ability to spread, the cells can wind up almost anywhere. The most common sites of spread include lymph nodes, lung, liver, skin, brain, spinal cord, and bone. When the malignant cells enter an organ they begin to multiply, forming individual tumors, and eventually they displace the normal cells. As time progresses, they will eventually interfere with the normal function of the organ, compromising the individuals' health. As the tumors become larger and more numerous, the functioning of the different organs of the body continue to deteriorate until the damage is overwhelming and the patients dies.

61. What are the symptoms that indicate that melanoma has metastasized?

The symptoms of metastatic melanoma depend on the site of spread. There are some general signs you should watch out for, including unexplained fatigue, a swelling in the skin or elsewhere, unexplained persistent pain, loss of appetite, or shortness of breath with or without cough. However, one of the major problems with developing metastatic disease in internal organs is that the tumors may grow quite large or there may be a significant number of them before symptoms become obvious. Therefore, if you're at high risk for recurrent disease, you should be aware of changes in your body, especially changes that become persistent and don't respond to attempts to alleviate them. It's important to bring these types of symptoms to the attention of your physician as early as possible. Site-specific symptoms are as follows:

If you're at high risk for recurrent disease, you should be aware of changes in your body.

Skin: Melanoma may spread to the skin in one of two fashions: intradermally or subcutaneously. In intradermal spread, melanoma cells are in the skin itself and appear as small black or pink dots. As they grow, they become more obvious, but they don't usually cause any symptoms unless they become quite large. Subcutaneous melanoma appears as a lump under the skin, usually without any color change. In some cases, the tumor may cause a blue or purple discoloration in the skin. This type of metastasis is usually pain-free, but if the metastasis occurs in the right location the pain may be significant. Metastatic lesions in bones or in areas that cause the liver to stretch may be particularly painful.

Lymph node: Tumor involvement of lymph nodes usually produces a lump that you can feel with or, more commonly, without pain. Obviously, the lump will appear in the lymph node group to which the tumor has metastasized. In some patients the physician may elect to have the tumor removed, while in other patients surgery is not indicated. Sites of common lymph node involvement include the neck, axilla, and the groin.

Lung: Early spread of melanoma to the lung may go undetected for a long period of time. If a patient is at high risk for metastatic disease, periodic CT and PET scans may detect a recurrent tumor long before any symptoms develop. Typical symptoms of lung tumors include chest heaviness; cough with or without sputum or blood; shortness of breath; fever; and, in some patients, pneumonia.

Liver: Again, early spread of melanoma to the liver is usually undetected and may be found by screening CT and PET scans. Symptoms include loss of appetite, nausea, vomiting, unexplained weight loss, jaundice (yellowing of the skin), unexplained fever, and pain in the right upper quadrant of the abdomen.

Bone: Spread to the bone is usually a late manifestation of metastatic disease, meaning that there is usually evidence of spread to other organs before the cancer appears in the bone. The most common symptom is pain over a bone. In some cases, a lump under the skin will also appear. If you notice these symptoms, you should contact your physician immediately. It's very important to determine if the spread has involved a weight-bearing bone such as the femur, the large bone in the thigh. Weight-bearing bones can be significantly weakened when a tumor has invaded. In this situation, it's not uncommon for bone to fracture with little or no trauma, a situation referred to as a pathologic fracture. If you're found to have a tumor in the bone, your physician may order a bone scan. This test may find very early tumors in the bones and can help direct your therapy. Treatment commonly involves radiation therapy to the area with the tumor. In some cases, it may be necessary to undergo a surgical procedure to stabilize the bone in order to prevent a fracture. Your physician should discuss the pros and cons of this approach with you.

Brain: Spread of melanoma to the brain is also usually a late complication of this disease. As with other internal sites, early spread to the brain may go unnoticed; however, because the brain is enclosed in the skull, there is not a lot of room for a tumor to grow. For this reason, brain tumors are usually found when they are small. One of the common responses of the brain to tumor invasion is the development of edema (swelling) around the tumor. In fact, it's common for such swelling to cause symptoms even when the tumor is small. Common symptoms include seizure (uncontrolled movements with or without loss of consciousness), headache, focal weakness (weakness in an arm or leg usually on the same side of the body), and personality change with or without confusion. The development of a brain tumor suggests a poor prognosis; however, new medicines and radiation therapy techniques have improved the outcome for some patients.

62. What treatment options do I have when the melanoma has spread?

Once melanoma has spread there are a variety of treatments that can be offered. To help choose the treatments that will ultimately be used, your physician will employ a complex decision pattern. You should be a partner in this decision-making process and fully understand why a particular treatment has been chosen. You're the one who must undergo the treatment, so you should understand the rationale behind the decision to use one mode of treatment over another. Also remember that the treatment plan may include more than one form of treatment.

Surgery

Generally, the first decision that is made is whether the disease can be removed surgically. There are a number of factors that are important in considering surgery, including location of the disease, the number of tumors present, and other medical problems that you may have. For example, removing a tumor from the lung may be appropriate for a 25-year-old healthy individual, but may make no sense at all for someone who is 75 years old with emphysema and heart disease. In the latter situation, surgery may kill the patient. Remember that surgery can only remove visible disease and will not treat microscopic disease that is hiding somewhere else. Therefore, some form of adjuvant or preventive therapy usually follows surgery in order to decrease the risk of further recurrence.

Radiation Therapy

Radiation therapy involves treatment with powerful particles that are generated using a radioactive source. A physician called a radiation oncologist usually administers this treatment. Similar to surgery, the radiation treats primarily disease that can be seen and some of the surrounding normal tissue. On occasion, radiation therapy is used to "sterilize" an area where a tumor has been removed—for example, if a tumor has been removed from a lymph node in the groin and there is evidence that the tumor grew outside of the lymph node. Radiation is commonly used when surgery isn't appropriate, such as in the treatment of an elderly patient who is otherwise not a surgical candidate.

Radiation is usually administered on a daily basis for between 1 and 6 weeks. Prior to starting the therapy, the area to be treated is "simulated" using special scans such as a CT scan. The treatment is planned and mapped out on the scan as well as the patient. The area to be treated is encompassed in a "port," which is the area that actually receives the radiation. It may be necessary to place pinhead-sized tattoos or mark the area with a long-lasting marker to define the port. The marks are used as guides to make sure that the rays of radiation are aimed correctly. In some cases "blocks" are designed to protect normal tissue and are used during each treatment. The blocks are made of lead or some other radiation-resistant material that prevents normal tissue from receiving any radiation. Additionally, the radiation oncologist must be careful of the different tolerances of normal tissue. Different tissues can absorb different total amounts of radiation. For instance, the spinal cord is more sensitive to radiation treatment than the lung. Therefore, if the spinal cord is to receive some of the radiation to be administered to an area, sometime prior to completion of the entire treatment the radiation oncologist may order the spinal cord to be blocked. The block gives the spinal cord protection while the remainder of the treatment is completed.

Immunotherapy

One of the curious things that we have known for a long time is that, under the right circumstances, the body's normal immune system can kill melanoma cells.

Radiation is commonly used when surgery isn't appropriate.

Under the right circumstances, the body's normal immune system can kill melanoma cells.

Treatment of Malignant Melanoma

The right circumstances at this time remain a mystery and are the subject of intense research. However, this insight has lead to the development of many different types of immunologically based treatments. These treatments range from directly injecting the tumor with immune activating agents such as **bacillus Calmette Guérin (BCG)** to using cytokines (proteins that activate the immune system) such as interleukin 2 (IL–2). Immunotherapy has been used in the adjuvant setting as well as in the treatment of established disease. This approach has also spawned the growing tumor vaccine biotherapy industry. In immunotherapy, the tumor cells are not killed directly by the agent that is given to the patient. Instead, the immunologic agent stimulates the production of immune cells that recognize cancer cells as abnormal. These immune cells can then kill malignant cells.

Bacillus Calmette Guérin (BCG)

The microorganism that causes a tuberculosis-like disease in cows. This organism can initiate a local immune response at the site of injection, which in some cases will result in local tumor destruction.

Chemotherapy

Chemotherapy is the treatment of cancer using medicines that can directly kill malignant cells. These medicines work through a variety of mechanisms to disrupt the normal function of the malignant cell. Unfortunately, the vast majority of these agents are not specific for malignant cells. Normal cells are also killed as a result of chemotherapy. The type of normal cells killed can depend on the specific chemotherapeutic agent used. For example, cisplatin is a chemotherapeutic agent that has detrimental effects on nerve cells but inflicts little damage on bone marrow cells. Doxorubicin, on the other hand, has little effect on nerves but significant effect on bone marrow cells. The fact that these two agents kill cancer cells but injure different types of normal cells allows physicians to use them together in what is called combination chemotherapy (using multiple chemotherapeutic agents at the same time). In fact, most cancers are treated with combination chemotherapy.

Some melanoma chemotherapy drugs are listed in Table 4. Not all drugs listed here are in general use for melanoma, although all have been approved by the FDA for other uses. Talk to your doctor about specific treatments.

Table 4   Commonly used agents to treat malignant melanoma

Drug Name Generic (Brand)	Maker	How Prescribed[1]
CHEMOTHERAPY		
Dacarbazine (DTIC®)	Bayer	FDA-approved for melanoma
Temozolomide (Temodar®)	Schering	Off-label; FDA-approved for brain tumors; in clinical trials for melanoma
Carboplatin (Paraplatin®)	Bristol-Myers	Off-label; in clinical trials for melanoma
Carmustine (BiCNU®)	Bristol-Myers	Off-label; in clinical trials for melanoma
Cisplatin (Platinol®)	Bristol-Myers	Off-label; in clinical trials for melanoma
Docetaxel (Taxotere®)	Aventis	Off-label; in clinical trials for melanoma
Lomustine (CeeNU®)	Bristol-Myers	Off-label; in clinical trials for melanoma
Thalidomide (Thalomid®)	Celgene	Off-label; in clinical trials for melanoma
Vinblastine (Velban®)	Eli Lilly and Co.	Off-label; in clinical trials for melanoma
IMMUNOTHERAPY		
Interferon-Alpha (Intron-A®)	Schering	FDA-approved as adjuvant therapy for malignant melanoma
Interleukin-2 (Proleukin®)	Chiron	FDA-approved for malignant melanoma
GM-CSF (Leukine®)	Immunex	Off-label; in clinical trials for melanoma
ANTI ESTROGEN		
Tamoxifen (Nolvadex®)	AstraZeneca	Off-label; in clinical trials for melanoma

[1]When the FDA approves a medication, it is generally approved for a given illness, such as breast cancer. It is common for medications used in cancer therapy to work in several different types of cancer in addition to the FDA-approved indication. Your oncologist may choose to use a medication for treating your melanoma even though there has not been FDA "approval" for this indication. This is acceptable practice and is allowed by law; however, some insurance companies will term this prescription "off label" use and decline coverage for its use.

Biochemotherapy

It has long been assumed that chemotherapeutic agents inhibit the immune response against malignant cells. However, several agents don't inhibit the immune system; they can actually enhance the immune response. This observation has lead to the development of biochemotherapy. In this approach, chemotherapy agents are administered in combination with agents that stimulate the immune system with the hope that the chemotherapeutic agents will directly attack the tumor cells while the immunologic agents stimulate an immune response. This approach has been shown to work mostly against malignant melanoma; however, clinical trials using this technique against other cancers are underway.

Targeted Therapy

One of the major benefits of all of the research that has been done over the last 40 years is the development of molecular biology. This is the branch of science that has allowed us to identify the specific proteins made by the abnormal genes that are in cancer cells. Using this information, physicians and scientists are working together to develop new agents that will target the specific abnormality in the cancer cell and initiate its destruction. It's hoped that the toxicity of the new agents will be limited as much as possible to the cancer cells. Although the research has not reached this point yet, there are new agents on the horizon that are creating great excitement. An example of a targeted therapy is the new agent referred to as STI–571, recently approved by the FDA under the brand name Gleevec. Leukemic cells in a specific type of leukemia called chronic myelogenous leukemia (CML) overproduce a specific enzyme that tells the leukemic cells to constantly divide, producing billions and billions of leukemic cells. STI–571 can turn off this enzyme, preventing the further production of these cancerous cells. While this agent still has side effects, many patients who previously would have died of their disease are now without any evidence of leukemia. The research that identified these new targets for attack may eventually help fight other types of cancer, including melanoma.

63. My melanoma has returned several times on the same leg. My doctor suggested that I undergo a limb perfusion. What is this?

When melanoma continues to come back on one of your limbs despite surgery and other attempts to control it, limb perfusion becomes a consideration. An isolated limb perfusion is a procedure that attempts to deliver a very high dose of chemotherapy or other form of treatment to the limb without it reaching other parts of the body.

During a limb perfusion the surgeon first surgically isolates the leg by placing catheters into the leg and placing a tourniquet on the leg to prevent leakage of the chemotherapy into the rest of the body. One of the catheters withdraws blood from the leg, transferring it to a machine that mixes in oxygen and the chemotherapy as it increases the temperature of the mixture. The other catheter returns the mixture to the leg. This procedure continues for up to an hour, after which the catheters are removed and the procedure is completed. This approach delivers a high concentration of chemotherapy to the tumor. The increased temperature seems to increase the uptake of the chemotherapy into the tumor cells themselves. The rest of the body receives very little of the chemotherapy, sparing it from the toxic effects of the treatment. Isolated limb perfusion is associated with local complications, sometimes including painful swelling of the leg along with nerve damage and, on occasion, breakdown of the skin. Most patients will recover nicely, but it may take several weeks.

64. What are the common side effects of treatment?

Obviously, the side effects that a patient experiences will depend upon the specific treatment that the individual receives. Additionally, the site that is treated also plays a role in some of the therapeutic interventions. Some general side effects are discussed below.

Surgery

The most common side effect of surgery is pain at the site of the surgery. This is due to the disruption of the normal tissue planes, inflammation that induces swelling of the tissue, and the disruption of normal nerve pathways. Pain is most difficult during the first 24 to 48 hours and subsequently improves each day. Depending on the severity of the pain, there are a variety of treatments that can be offered. In cases where the surgery involves a small area, taking oral pain medication can usually control pain. In come cases, nonnarcotic medications such as acetaminophen or ibuprofen are sufficient. However, narcotic medications such as acetaminophen plus codeine or hydrocodone are commonly needed. In severe cases, morphine or one of its derivatives such as hydromorphine is used.

If the surgical procedure involves entering a major body cavity such as the thorax (chest) or abdomen, narcotic pain medications that can be infused intravenously are used in the immediate 24- to 72-hour postoperative period. The intravenous medications are subsequently changed to oral medications when you're able to tolerate them.

On occasion, despite all attempts to keep an area sterile, the surgical wound may develop an infection. In this situation, antibiotics administered either intravenously or orally are started in an attempt to kill the invading organism. If the infection is deep, it may be necessary to open the wound and drain the infected material.

Finally, you must prepare yourself for the cosmetic effect of the surgery, especially if the area operated on is highly visible such as an area on the face. On occasion, the initial procedure results in some amount of disfigurement that will ultimately require reconstructive surgery. Surgeons may elect to delay the reconstructive procedure until the tissue is less inflamed. Alternatively, the procedure may need to be done in a stepwise fashion, requiring two or more procedures. It's important to prepare yourself emotionally for this event.

You must prepare yourself for the cosmetic effect of the surgery.

Radiation Therapy

The most common side effect of radiation therapy is inflammation of the skin in the area that is irradiated. This inflammation may appear similar to sunburn, or may develop to the point where the skin breaks down, resulting in the loss of skin. In most cases the skin heals with some help from antibiotic creams. In the most serious cases, surgery may be necessary.

Depending on the area radiated, normal tissue may also be treated. The radiation therapist will take precautions to limit the damage to these tissues, but some damage is inevitable. The resulting symptoms will be site dependent. For example, if the esophagus (swallowing tube) is involved it may become very painful to swallow food or drink. If the bladder is involved, urination may become compromised. It's therefore critically important for you to discuss this issue with your radiation oncologist so that you can be prepared for any complication that results from treatment.

Immunotherapy

There are many different immunotherapy medications currently in use, but they all tend to have similar side effects. In most cases, patients experience what are described as "flu-like" symptoms, such as fever, chills, muscle pain (**myalgias**), joint pain (**arthralgias**), dermatitis (skin rash), nausea, vomiting, and diarrhea. Frequently, the fever can reach as high as 104°F and can be associated with rigors (uncontrollable shaking chills). The medications most commonly associated with the above symptoms include interferon and interleukin–2. There are a variety of interventions that can be used to deal with the side effects of the medications. You should discuss such interventions with your physician before you start therapy.

Chemotherapy

The side effects of chemotherapy vary widely depending on the agent involved. Specific agents are discussed below. Since chemotherapy medications usually kill rapidly dividing cells, there are some predictable side

Myalgias

An inflammation of the muscles that causes pain or an ache within the muscle.

Arthralgias

An inflammation of one or more joints that causes pain (usually without swelling). The joints may feel stiff, and it's usually painful to bend the affected joint.

effects that occur. The gastrointestinal (GI) tract has a lining that is continually replacing itself, so it's a common site for problems. A side effect called mucositis (inflamed mucous membranes) can occur in the mouth. In mucositis, the lining cells of the mouth are killed, resulting in a breakdown of the lining. Painful sores then develop in the mouth, which can make eating problematic. The extent of this side effect can range from mild discomfort to a complete inability to eat, which requires using an alternative means of obtaining nutrition. A similar situation in the esophagus is called esophagitis, which makes swallowing next to impossible. Such breakdown in the stomach or intestines can result in abdominal pain and, in severe cases, bleeding. If breakdown occurs in the rectum, severe diarrhea and bleeding may occur. In general, these symptoms will last from 3 to 10 days depending on the severity of the damage.

Nausea and vomiting are common side effects and may occur without any overt evidence of damage. There are a variety of strategies that are used to deal with these side effects. In most cases, antinausea medications are administered in an attempt to prevent symptoms before they start. The newest medications have significantly improved the ability to control this side effect. However, there are still patients in whom nausea and vomiting are problematic. For these patients, multiple medication changes are necessary to find an effective agent.

Hair loss is a common side effect of many chemotherapeutic agents. To date, there is no effective means to prevent it. If hair loss occurs, the hair almost always returns. Nevertheless, few side effects cause more concern for patients. In many ways, hair loss declares the patient's illness to the world, causing more emotional distress than any other side effect. Hair appliances are available to provide a sense of control for patients so inclined.

Jodie's comment:

I was lucky not to lose my hair with the chemo—although it did make me sick! You get terrible body aches, fevers in the evenings, a metallic taste in your mouth, which makes food taste bad, sometimes mouth sores, a tired and run-down feeling, and loss of appetite, among other things. Actually, it was difficult to eat. I had to figure out what foods were easy to swallow, such as soup and scrambled eggs. And through all of this, I was constantly nauseous (I ate half of a roll of Rolaids before it dawned on me that this was nausea).

I realized that I felt terrible no matter what I did whether I was sitting on the couch or lying in bed, neither of which I wanted to do. So I went to work. I was lucky to be working for my boyfriend's family so I could come and go, as I needed. I usually didn't get sick until a little later in the day, around 3:00 p.m. or so. Someone would give me a ride home before then. Not only did I get physical symptoms; I also got mental symptoms. I felt bored and lonely. It really helped to have an agenda for the day. I went through this cycle three times. Each time you feel worse than the last one.

Well, here I am. I made it!! It's been three years since my cancer was removed. I am still cancer free!! My 30th birthday was last weekend and I couldn't be happier that I am turning over a new leaf in my life.

PART SEVEN

Clinical Trials

What is a clinical trial?

How do I find out about clinical trials?

What are the different types of clinical trials?

More ...

65. What is a clinical trial?

The unsung heroes who participate in clinical trials fight the war against cancer on a daily basis. Every day thousands of patients agree to enter clinical trials that test new medications or new combinations of medications so their effectiveness can be determined. Many advances have been made that will benefit the individuals who develop cancer in the future because these patients and their families participated in clinical trials. Enough cannot be said about the courage of these individuals.

There are many people who are afraid to enter a clinical trial because they don't want to be a "guinea pig." Nothing is further from the truth! Everyone who is offered the opportunity to enter a clinical trial has the right to refuse to participate and therefore makes a conscious decision. However, those who choose to enter clinical trials have a different attitude. Almost every individual who enters a clinical trial does so with the attitude, "If it doesn't help me, maybe it will help someone else." In the words of Sam Moss from Calhoun, Georgia, just one of these many heroes involved in clinical trials, "I would enter any clinical trial if it leads to something that will prevent one of my children or grandchildren from having to face this disease."

In general, clinical trials are designed to test a new medication or combination of medications in specific patient populations. The various types of clinical trials will be discussed below. All clinical trials require that patients understand the purpose of the trial and patients must voluntarily agree to participate. This freedom of choice is imperative and is the foundation of any trial.

Clinical Trials

The first step in a clinical trial involves the physician developing a question or situation to be tested. For example, the trial may be designed to test a new cancer drug in patients with melanoma. Once the question or situation to be investigated is identified, the protocol, under which the trial will be conducted, is written. This protocol describes the rationale for the trial as well as the rules governing who is eligible and how the treatment is to be given. The protocol also contains the consent form that participants will be required to sign. The consent form provides participants with specific information about the conduct of the trial that is required by law. The consent form is necessary for any trial that involves human subjects.

After the protocol is completed, it's sent to an Institutional Review Board (IRB) composed of individuals who have no vested interest in the trial. These individuals evaluate the scientific design of the trial, ensure that there are safety measures to protect the participants, and ensure that the consent form is clearly written and easily understood. If the IRB approves the trial, it can begin.

If you are asked to participate in a clinical trial, make sure that you understand the purpose of the trial and what you'll be asked to do. Don't be afraid to ask questions. It's important that you feel comfortable with the intent of the trial and your role in it. After all of your questions have been answered, you'll be asked to sign the consent form. Read it completely and ask any final questions before you sign the document. It's important to always remember that even though the physician directs the trial, *you* decide whether or not to participate or continue to participate after you have started

If you are asked to participate in a clinical trial, make sure that you understand the purpose of the trial and what you'll be asked to do.

the trial. If after entering a clinical trial you decide that you don't want to continue, you have every right to stop at any time.

The success of clinical trials may be best exemplified by studies conducted in treating women with breast cancer. Twenty years ago almost every woman with breast cancer underwent a radical mastectomy. There was evidence to suggest that removing only the tumor (lumpectomy) and then treating the breast with radiation could treat women with small tumors (4 cm or less). In order to answer the question, "Is the survival of these two groups of women the same?" a large clinical trial was conducted randomizing hundreds of women between treatment with radical mastectomy or lumpectomy plus radiation. Through the courage of these women, the answer was obtained. It's now known that either approach is effective, and women have the choice of which treatment to undergo. As a result, many hundreds of thousands of women have opted for the less radical procedure, preserving their breast. These women have benefited directly from the information obtained from this trial.

66. How do I find out about clinical trials?

Despite the fact that there are thousands of clinical trials available, only about 3% of cancer patients participate. This is one of the great tragedies of cancer care today. If you're interested in participating in clinical trials, you should begin by asking your physician if your clinic or hospital participates in the conduct of clinical trials. While clinical trials historically have been conducted primarily at university centers, today cutting edge cancer research is occurring in independent cancer centers located in communities across the United States. This provides more patients access to many new forms of treatment. It will decrease the amount of time it takes to finish a trial and obtain the answers needed to advance cancer care. If your physician doesn't participate in clinical trials, contact the National Cancer Institute's Cancer Information Service at 1–800–4-CANCER. Additionally, web sites such as the National Cancer Institute's clinical trial site *www.cancer.gov/clinical_trials* and the National Institute of Health site *www.clinicaltrials.gov* are also valuable sources of information. Finally, there are many cancer-type-specific sites that are managed by patients, such as the Melanoma Patients Information Page (*www.mpip.org*), that provide useful information.

67. What are the different types of clinical trials?

For the most part there are three basic types of clinical trials: Phase I, II, and III. Phase I trials are generally conducted to determine how much of a medication can be safely given and how the human body metabolizes the drug. These trials represent the initial study of the drug in humans. Usually, no more than 20 to 50 volunteers are needed to complete the study. Side effects of the drug are typically associated with higher doses. Similarly, the effectiveness of a particular drug will usually increase with higher doses. Successful completion of a phase I trial will lead to a phase II trial.

Phase II trials are designed to obtain information regarding the effectiveness of a new drug for specific uses (indications). Several hundred volunteers may be enrolled in a number of phase II studies that are conducted concurrently involving several different types of tumors. If phase II trials identify activity of a new agent when used alone, the next step may be studies that test the results of the addition of the new medication to a more standard regimen. Otherwise the new medication may go onto phase III trials.

Phase III trials are studies that are designed to determine the effectiveness of a new treatment against what is considered the standard treatment. In some cases, there is no standard therapy. Instead, the treatment may be tested against a placebo (an agent that has no medicinal value) or an untreated group of patients. The group of patients who receive the standard treatment is called the control group. The individuals receiving the new medicine make up the test or study group. Phase III studies are often referred to as randomized double-blind controlled trials. This means that the physician has no control over which treatment the patient receives. The physician and the patient are unaware of which treatment the patient actually receives. In non-blinded randomized trials, the treatment is known, but the physician has no control over which treatment the patient receives. The goal of phase III trials is to compare the overall benefit of the standard treatment against the overall benefit of the investigational treatment. Depending on the needs of the study, several hundred to several thousand volunteers may be enrolled in the study.

68. Does treatment on a clinical trial cost me money?

Clinical trials are funded in different ways and much depends upon who is the trial sponsor. In the setting of a trial sponsored by the National Cancer Institute, funding may be provided to cover the cost of the entire treatment. This is especially true if the agent being tested is brand new and has never been given to patients. In this case, you may be asked to stay overnight in the hospital so that the physicians can take blood tests to determine how your body metabolized the drug. This is referred to as a pharmacokinetic study.

Cooperative groups run many trials. In this setting, physicians from various institutions and areas of the country agree to conduct the same trial to allow more individuals to access it. Additionally, this strategy helps to obtain the required number of patients faster than if the study is done at only one place. Cooperative group trials may not fund the entire treatment. Sometimes the trial involves adding a new medication to a standard regimen of medications. The study may cover the cost of the new medication, but may ask you or your insurance company to pay for the standard treatment.

In some cases a pharmaceutical company that is testing one of its new agents sponsors the study. Generally, the pharmaceutical company will cover the cost of the treatment and any ancillary issues.

Finally, there are situations in which individual physicians begin a type of trial that is referred to as an investigator-initiated trial. In this type of trial there may not be any funding. This type of trial typically uses medications that are already approved, but uses them as part of a new combination. You or your insurance company may be asked to pay for this treatment. In most cases, this treatment will include agents that should be covered by your insurance; however, it's always important to check this out before you begin treatment.

69. *What are the major risks and benefits of being in a clinical trial?*

Jodie's comment:

There is only one risk that I can think of, and that's the "sense of the unknown." You are involved with testing new treatments and sometimes the effects of the treatment are unknown. Your experience is documented and compared with others treated on your trial. It was comforting to know that there were other people are going through this at the same time. One of the major benefits was being involved in testing new treatments that might improve your chances of surviving, and also the information learned may be helpful to the next person.

In general, clinical trials are conducted to answer an important question in the treatment of patients in a particular clinical situation. They are designed first and foremost with the safety of the participant in mind. Under no circumstances should a trial be designed that knowingly compromises the treatment of the patient. If there is a treatment that offers a chance for cure, the investigational treatment must have at least an equivalent response rate in order for the trial to go forward. However, it's very important that you discuss the purpose of the clinical trial with your physician and understand the other treatments that you might consider.

To some degree, the major risks that you take participating in a clinical trial are related to the phase of the study that you're entering. In phase I trials, either a new medicine is being tested for which there is little experience using it in humans, or there is a new combination of medicines being tested and safe doses of the various medicines need to be identified. In this type of trial, little may be known about safe doses or side effects, so unknown side effects are a potential risk. Additionally, unexpected medication interactions may occur that may be either harmful or beneficial. Sometimes the combination of medications may increase the risk of toxicity. However, there have also been situations in which new combinations proved to be more effective than expected because of a previously unknown interaction. In general, it's safe to say that phase I trials pose the most risk to the patient as far as the potential to develop toxic side effects.

During phase II trials, the doses and side effects of the medications used are pretty much known. There are usually few unknown risks. The same is true in phase III trials. However, in phase III trials the issue of randomization must be considered. In a phase III trial that includes a placebo group, you may be randomized to the placebo group and therefore receive no therapy. A placebo group is only used when there is no known effective therapy. If the trial includes a placebo group, it will be identified in the consent form.

There are a number of benefits associated with treatment in clinical trials. In most cases, clinical trials are testing either new medications or combinations of medications for which there is experimental evidence to suggest that a positive benefit may be expected. You will have access to cutting edge treatments not available to the general public. Treatment is usually administered at centers that have significant experience in the conduct of clinical trials. Finally, by entering a clinical trial you have the opportunity to contribute to medical knowledge.

70. Who is eligible for treatment in a clinical trial?

The principal investigator of the study and the type of trial that is being offered determine all the answers to the above questions. The investigator determines which patients are eligible for the trial. In some trials any patient with cancer is eligible. In other cases, the trial may be restricted to patients with a particular form of cancer. When the actions of the medication are known, the investigator may anticipate certain potential complications and restrict entry into the trial to patients without certain medical conditions. For example, the use of immune system stimulating agents is frequently associated with fluid accumulation in the lungs. This could put certain patients, such as those with a history of heart disease, at risk for severe complications, potentially even death. In this situation, it's appropriate to exclude patients with known heart disease from the trial.

71. How long will the trial last, and what will be required of me? Can I be in more than one clinical trial at a time?

How long a trial lasts depends on the type of trial being conducted. For instance, a phase I trial that is testing a new medicine may be over in a matter of weeks for some patients, while a patient on a phase III trial may expect to be followed for years. It's important for you to have the duration of the trial clarified before you agree to enter it.

In most cases, the clinical trial is administered to patients close to their homes. However, certain trials are only available at specific institutions, such as the National Cancer Institute. Patients may be required to travel to the institution.

In general, a patient can only participate in one trial at a time. The purpose of the clinical trial is to test the efficacy of a particular treatment. If you were to receive more than one treatment at a time it would be impossible to determine which treatment worked (if any). For this reason you will be restricted from entering more than one trial at a time. If one of the trials doesn't include treatment, then it's possible to be on two trials at the same time. In some cases, a treatment protocol will have a "Quality of Life" companion protocol where one of the protocols simply requires the patient to answer questions about how he or she is tolerating the treatment. In this situation, it's acceptable to be on both protocols at the same time.

It's common to be on consecutive protocols wherein the patient is offered treatment on a second protocol if the first treatment doesn't work. However, the investigator must be sure that the patient has recovered from the first treatment and that the treatment's effectiveness has been determined.

PART EIGHT

Non-Melanoma Skin Cancers

What is an actinic keratosis?

What do actinic keratoses look like?

What are the risk factors associated with the development of AKs?

More . . .

72. What is an actinic keratosis?

Actinic keratosis

A lesion of the skin that is induced by UV radiation from the sun. It typically appears as a small (2–10 mm) erythematous scaling lesion on a sun exposed area of the body. It is a pre-malignant lesion, i.e., it has the potential to become malignant.

Actinic keratoses (AKs) are commonly thought to represent premalignant lesions that, given enough time, will ultimately turn into cancer. AKs are caused by long-term exposure to UV rays found in the sun. Historically, AKs typically appeared in patients ages 40–50 after years of chronic exposure to the sun. However, recent data have demonstrated that AKs are now commonly found in individuals in their teens and twenties who are from geographic areas with year-round high-intensity sunlight, such as Florida and southern California. In patients with fair skin living in areas of high sun exposure the incidence of AKs is over 50%.

Under the microscope skin cells (keratinocytes) found in the epidermis that are altered in size and shape characterize AKs. Typically, there is an alteration in the appearance of the nucleus. This alteration, referred to as dysplasia, can extend deeper into the second layer of the skin, the dermis. These cells tend to cluster together and spread horizontally in the skin without penetrating deeper than the dermis.

73. What do actinic keratoses look like?

The appearance of the skin that is associated with UV damage can be very subtle initially. AKs typically begin as a small (2–3 mm) area of redness that may easily be overlooked. However, as time progresses, the area of redness doesn't heal and usually becomes noticeable. Still many people don't realize that this lesion may be a precursor to the development of a skin cancer.

With the passage of more time, the lesion will usually develop a dry, scale-like surface and feel rough to the touch (Plate 8). Although they usually have a reddish base they also can appear to be flesh-colored, reddish brown, or even yellow in color. They may be as small as 2 to 3 mm but can achieve any size and shape frequently with very irregular borders. Most commonly they are flat with the surface of the skin, but on occasion they will be elevated a few millimeters. There are usually surprisingly few symptoms with these lesions, although some patients report that the lesion itches or bleeds a small amount. Wrinkling and furrowing of the skin, which are other manifestations of UV damage, may be present in conjunction with AK lesions.

74. What are the risk factors associated with the development of AKs?

Factors associated with the development of AKs are similar to those associated with the development of melanoma. These factors include fair skin and limited tanning ability. The duration and frequency of UV exposure as well as the intensity of the exposure are also important factors in the development of these lesions.

75. How are AKs diagnosed?

Their clinical appearance and the history given by the patient most commonly identify AKs. A flat, red, scaling lesion in a patient who burns easily and doesn't tan well is most likely an AK. Given this, it's common for these lesions to be treated without first doing a biopsy. In most cases, this is a perfectly safe and effective approach. However, if there is any question about the identity of the lesion, a biopsy should be performed.

76. How are AKs treated?

AKs are most commonly treated using some form of topical treatment. It's unusual to employ systemic treatments. The most common treatments include the following:

Cryosurgery: This is the most common form of treatment. Liquid nitrogen is used to freeze the lesion. Immediately after treatment a small red blister forms and the area becomes mildly painful. The frozen tissue ultimately recovers and the healing process results in the development of normal skin in the treated area.

Surgical excision and biopsy: At times, it may be difficult to be sure that the lesion in question is not a more serious skin cancer. In this situation the lesion is best treated by surgical removal. The pathologist then evaluates the material.

Topical and systemic retinoids: Vitamin A and its derivatives are strong agents that can normalize the growth of cells that have been damaged by UV radiation. These agents can be administered either as a cream applied directly to the skin or taken internally. These medications are associated with a number of side effects and commonly result in skin irritation.

Topical chemotherapy: The chemotherapy agent 5-fluorouracil has been found to attack AKs, which results in their replacement with normal skin. This agent was originally developed as an intravenous medication, but it has been reformulated into a cream for direct application to the lesion of concern.

Chemical peel: This treatment involves applying irritating chemical agents to the skin. As part of the healing process, the damaged skin blisters and peels, and is replaced by normal skin. This approach results in irritated appearing skin with significant redness.

Dermabrasion: Rapidly rotating brushes wear away the skin, removing layers of UV-damaged skin. New skin grows to replace the damaged skin.

Laser skin resurfacing: Carbon dioxide lasers are used to burn damaged tissue, allowing new skin to appear.

Electrosurgical skin resurfacing: This approach uses electromagnetic energy to remove the damaged layer of skin. New skin will surface to replace the removed tissue.

It's important to protect new skin from additional UV damage. Liberal use of sunscreens and moisturizers is an important part of caring for recovering skin.

77. Why do AKs represent a health risk?

AKs are not generally symptomatic, except for occasional itching. However, there's a risk that these lesions can degenerate and become squamous cell carcinomas, so they require attention. The treatment of these lesions costs many millions of dollars each year, representing a significant portion of the cost of health care today.

78. Do AKs become melanoma?

No! Other than the fact that AKs are also observed in patients with melanoma because they share common risk factors, there is no direct relationship between AKs and melanoma.

79. I have a cutaneous horn. What is this, and is it dangerous?

On rare occasions, the UV-damaged skin cells are stimulated to grow into a lesion that resembles the horn of an animal, hence its name "cutaneous horn." This lesion is almost always found on sun-exposed skin, typically on the ear. The lesion will continue to grow unless it's removed. It can become large and assume either a straight, curved, or twisted shape. Cutaneous horns deserve attention as early as possible because they occur in UV-damaged areas and carry the potential for malignant degeneration.

80. What is a basal cell carcinoma?

Basal cell carcinomas (BCCs) are malignant lesions of the skin that are the result of UV-induced damage in the basal cells, the cells located at the base of the epidermis. These cells don't form keratin. They remain at the basal layer for the majority of their natural history. BCCs are the most common cancer in the United States, accounting for 75% of all non-melanoma skin cancers and almost 25% of all cancers today.

81. What does a basal cell carcinoma look like?

Most BCCs appear as a reddened, raised lesion that is round or oval (Plate 2). BCCs take on a pearly sheen when a light is shined directly on them. They frequently have dilated blood vessels (telangiectasia) that occasionally bleed into the lesion, appearing as a small area of bleeding. Less frequently, BCCs appear much like an AK; a rough reddened scaling area on a sun-exposed surface of the skin.

82. Where are BCCs commonly found on the skin?

BCCs are slightly more common in men than women, and occur most frequently on sun-exposed skin. Of interest, approximately 30% of these lesions are found on the nose. These lesions used to be uncommon in individuals under the age of 50. However, with the marked increase in UV exposure at younger ages, BCCs are now commonly found in individuals younger than 50.

83. Can you inherit BCCs?

Yes, there are several instances in which BCCs are inherited. Recent studies have identified a gene referred to as the PTCH (patch) gene. This gene is inherited in a syndrome called nevoid basal cell carcinoma syndrome. The PTCH gene has also been found to be abnormal in patients who develop BCCs in a non-inherited fashion. There are several additional syndromes in which abnormal genes have yet to be identified.

84. Are there different types of basal cell cancers?

There are basically three different types of BCCs including:

- *Nodular:* The most common form appears as a pearly dome shaped lesion. On occasion these lesions may be pigmented and are difficult to differentiate from malignant melanoma. In this case it's imperative that a biopsy be performed because the surgical treatment is much different.

- *Superficial:* This form of BCC appears as a flat, scaling, reddened area that is difficult to differentiate from an AK. These lesions are also misdiagnosed as benign lesions such as **eczema** and **psoriasis**. Again, a biopsy is needed to make the diagnosis.
- *Morphea:* This form of BCC presents as a flat, slightly firm lesion without clear borders. It's sometimes mistaken for a scar. Morphea may appear to be undermining the skin, producing heaped-up areas of skin.

Eczema

An allergic reaction of the skin that appears as an area of redness, occasionally with small bumps, that frequently itches. The area frequently develops rough and dry skin overlying the reddened area.

Psoriasis

A chronic condition of the skin characterized by plaque-like areas of red, inflamed skin that commonly itches. The lesions can appear anywhere on the body but can frequently be found in areas where the skin bends, such as around the elbows.

85. How is a basal cell carcinoma treated?

The treatments used for AKs are often used to treat BCCs. However, it's much more common for BCCs to be treated using some form of surgical procedure so that a biopsy can be performed to diagnose suspected cancer. Most BCCs will not be life threatening, but they can be quite a bit larger than they appear and require a large amount of tissue to be removed to get the entire lesion. Mohs' micrographic surgery is commonly used to remove these lesions, especially in areas such as the face, so the surgeon can limit the amount of normal tissue that is removed.

86. Do basal cell carcinomas metastasize?

These lesions almost never metastasize. However, they can undermine large areas of what appears to be normal skin, and require extensive surgery to remove them in their entirety. In particular, the morphea form of this disease can be difficult to manage. Local recurrences can be devastating in areas such as the nose and eyes, when complete removal may require the surgical removal of the involved organ.

87. What is a squamous cell carcinoma?

Squamous cell carcinomas (SCCs) are cancers of the skin that develop from the cells of the epidermis that produce keratin. Like BCCs, SCCs are more common in men than women and represent the second most common human malignancy after BCCs. Many of the risk factors for developing this disease are the same as those for melanoma and BCCs, including patients taking immunosuppressive medications and patients with psoriasis treated with psoralen and UVA light. Finally, patients exposed to arsenic have an increased incidence of SCCs, especially Bowen's disease (see Question 90).

88. What do these lesions look like?

As with most skin cancers, SCCs are found in areas of the skin that have increased sun exposure. SCCs typically present as slightly raised, red, thick lesions that are dull in appearance, and commonly ulcerate and bleed (Plate 3). It may be difficult to distinguish these lesions from AKs, BCCs, benign lesions such as seborrheic keratosis, and inflammatory lesions.

89. Are SCCs inherited?

In most cases, SCCs are similar to BCCs in that they occur in patients who inherit an inability to tan well. Individuals with inherited syndromes, such as xeroderma pigmentosum and albinism, are at a higher risk for developing this disease. Additionally, SCCs are common in areas of chronically damaged skin, such as areas of radiation, burn scars, chronic inflammatory dermatoses, ulcers, and bone infections.

90. What are the different types of SCCs?

There are several types of SCC, including:

- *SCC in situ:* This is an SCC that has not invaded beyond the epidermis.
- *Invasive SCC:* This lesion has invaded into the dermis and carries a higher incidence of metastasis.
- *Bowen's disease:* This form of SCC in situ has a particular appearance under the microscope. This is the most common form of SCC in patients exposed to arsenic.
- *Erythroplasia of Queyrat:* Bowen's disease of the penis.
- *Keratoacanthomas:* SCCs of the skin that tend to form ulcerated, dome-shaped lesions. These SCCs are characterized by rapid initial growth followed by stabilization and ultimately spontaneous regression without active treatment.

91. How are SCCs treated?

SCCs are treated similarly to BCCs. However, because of the higher propensity for this form of skin cancer to metastasize, it's imperative that it be removed in its entirety. Non-surgical approaches should only be used when there is great confidence in the diagnosis and the likelihood that the area of concern is a superficial lesion. Radiation therapy is also used frequently if lesions are on areas such as the lips and around the eyes.

92. Do SCCs metastasize?

Lesions that invade the lower levels of the skin have a propensity to recur locally and may cause significant problems with local control. Unlike BCCs, SCCs metastasize at a higher rate to regional lymph nodes and internal organs. This is a particular problem in patients with an underlying immunosuppressive disorder.

Invasive SCCs metastasize at a rate of 3%–5%. This risk is increased when the area involved is a mucosal surface such as the lip, or an area of prior injury (scars, chronic ulcers). Additionally, invasive lesions on the mid-face or lip have the potential to involve local nerves, producing significant pain.

SCCs arising in an area of chronic inflammation metastasize at a rate of 10% to 30%, in contrast to those in noninflammatory sites that have a rate of 0.05% to 16%.

93. What is a Merkel cell carcinoma?

A Merkel cell carcinoma is a rare skin cancer that arises from cells in the skin called neuroendocrine cells. These tumors tend to behave aggressively and metastasize to a variety of areas including lymph nodes and other internal organs. These tumors are treated aggressively from initial diagnosis, frequently requiring the use of radiation and/or systemic chemotherapy. This disease carries a high mortality rate if it's not cured by surgical removal.

94. What is Kaposi's sarcoma?

Kaposi's sarcoma (KS) is a malignancy of cells in the skin called vascular endothelial cells. These cells make up the blood vessels that provide nutrients to the skin. KS is characterized by flat, violet colored patches of skin that grow together into nodules (masses) that can be quite large. As time progresses, the lesions can develop thick skin-like covering or break down and ulcerate.

95. Are there different forms of KS?

There are several types of KS, including:

- *Classic:* This form of KS occurs most commonly in elderly men of Ashkenazi Jewish or Mediterranean descent. It's characterized by the appearance of KS lesions that are located primarily on the lower extremities. These lesions are slow growing and slowly progress up the leg.
- *African endemic:* This form is further divided into a form of benign nodular growth found in young adults, and an aggressive disease that invades the lymph nodes of young children with great severity.
- *Iatrogenic:* This form of KS is seen in patients who have been taking immunosuppressive medications for a prolonged period of time. This disease may spontaneously regress when the medication is discontinued.
- *AIDS-related:* This form of KS is seen in patients with full-blown AIDS and is generally very aggressive. It's commonly responsible for the death of the patient.

96. How is KS treated?

Indolent forms of KS (forms that cause little or no pain and progress slowly) are generally treated with surgical excision or topical retinoid therapy. The slow growth of the disease allows for patients and physicians to try different treatments if the first approach is unsuccessful. More aggressive forms require systemic treatment with agents such as interferons and chemotherapeutic agents.

97. What is a lymphoma?

Lymphomas are cancers of cells that are called **lymphocytes**. Lymphocytes are white blood cells that participate in the immune response of the body. These cells are called either B or T cells. Particular T cells have a tendency to spread to the skin causing a disease called cutaneous T-cell lymphoma. Plaque-like, reddish lesions that can grow together and become very large characterize this disease. They may elevate off the surface of the skin and become quite disfiguring. As the disease progresses, the malignant cells may also involve the lymph nodes, and are sometimes found in the blood.

Lymphocytes
White blood cells that function in the bodies natural defense against viruses, bacteria, and cancer cells.

98. How are lymphomas treated?

Treatment for lymphomas of the skin depends on the stage of the disease (how extensively the disease has spread). Involvement of the skin is usually treated with topical chemotherapy, UVA phototherapy, injections of interferon, and local radiation therapy. Involvement of the lymph nodes or blood will require treatment with systemic therapy such as interferons, retinoids (derivatives of vitamin A), antibodies, and systemic chemotherapy.

99. Do cancers that start in other areas of the body ever show up in the skin?

The skin is a common site of metastasis from other types of cancer. The most common cancers to metastasize to the skin include breast, colon, and melanoma in

Non-Melanoma Skin Cancers

women and lung, colon, and melanoma in men. Other malignancies to involve the skin include cancers of the kidney, ovary, and stomach. Although metastatic lesions can occur in any area, the scalp (possibly because of its rich blood supply) is a very common site.

100. Where can I get more information?

This book can't provide comprehensive answers to all questions about skin cancer and melanoma. However, the Appendix that follows lists many organizations, web sites, and books that are reliable resources for accurate and up-to-date information. Note that web sites listed in the Appendix are up-to-date as of November 2002, but some may have changed; if you cannot reach the site listed here, use a web search engine (Google, Altavista, Lycos, Yahoo, etc.) to locate the site.

General Resources: Organizations

Non-profit Cancer or Dermatological Organizations

American Academy of Dermatology (AAD)
1350 I Street NW, Suite 880
Washington, DC 20005–4355
Phone: 202–842–3555
Web site: *www.aad.org*

American Cancer Society (ACS)
American Cancer Society National Home Office
1599 Clifton Road
Atlanta, GA 30329
Phone: 800–ACS–2345
Web site: *www.cancer.org*
Provides a wealth of information about treatments, prevention, and detection for
all forms of cancer.

American Melanoma Foundation
3914 Murphy Canyon Road, Suite A132
San Diego, CA 92123
Phone: 858–277–4426
Web site: *www.melanomafoundation.org*

American Society of Clinical Oncology (ASCO)
1900 Duke Street, Suite 200
Alexandria, VA 22314
Phone: 703–299–0150
Web site: *www.asco.org* or *www.peoplelivingwithcancer.org*
The American Society of Clinical Oncology represents 18,000 cancer profes-
sionals worldwide. The Society offers scientific and educational programs and

a wide range of other initiatives intended to foster the exchange of information about cancer. A section of the website is dedicated to "People Living with Cancer" (Web site: *www.people-livingwithcancer.org*) and provides information on cancer prevention and treatment, and other useful resources, such as online discussion groups and specific information on types of oncologists and tips on how to select the best oncologist for you.

Association of Cancer Online Resources (ACOR)
173 Duane Street, Suite 3A
New York NY 10013–3334
Phone: 212–226–5525
Web site: *www.acor.org*
Non-profit organization providing access to online cancer support groups and mailing lists for specific cancers.

Cancer Care, Inc.
275 7th Avenue
New York, NY 10001
Phone: 212–712–8400 (administration); 212–712–8080 (services)
Web site: *www.cancercare.org*
Provides online support groups for patients and families. Special section on melanoma.

National Comprehensive Cancer Network
50 Huntingdon Pike, Suite 200
Rockledge, PA 19046
Phone: 888–909–NCCN
Web site: *www.nccn.org*
This site provides information about cancer treatment centers around the U.S. It gives specific information regarding the institutions and their specialties, facilities, and resources. The site also provides cancer treatment guidelines specifically written for the patient.

National Coalition for Skin Cancer Prevention
c/o American Association for Health Education
1900 Association Drive
Reston, Virginia 20191
Phone: 703–476–3427
Web site: *www.sunsafety.org*
Provides basic information about sun safety and skin cancer prevention.

San Diego Melanoma Research Center
910 Sycamore Avenue, Suite 102
Vista, CA 92083
Web site: *www.sdcri.org*

Skin Cancer Foundation
245 5th Avenue, Suite 1403
New York, NY 10016
General Phone Inquiries: 800–SKIN–490
Web site: *www.skincancer.org*
National and international organization dedicated to providing information related exclusively to skin cancer.

Government Agencies

Centers for Disease Control and Prevention (CDC)
1600 Clifton Road
Atlanta, GA 30333
Phone: 404–639–3534 / 800–311–3435
Web site: *www.cdc.gov*

Centers for Medicaid and Medicare Services
Web site: *www.cms.hhs.gov*
Provides extensive information on Medicaid and Medicare, including information on referrals, individual state plans, and how to apply.

Health Resources and Services Administration (HRSA)
Hill-Burton Program
U.S. Department of Health and Human Services
Parklawn Building
5600 Fishers Lane
Rockville, MD 20857
Phone: 301–443–5656 / 800–638–0742 / 800–492–0359 (if calling from the Maryland area)
Web site: *www.hrsa.gov/osp/dfcr/about/aboutdiv.htm*
Under the U.S. Department of Health and Human Services, the HRSA provides information on many government initiatives and programs related to providing health care to low income and disadvantaged populations.

National Cancer Institute (NCI)
Cancer Information Service/CancerNet
Office of Cancer Communications
31 Center Drive
Building 31, Rm 10A07
Bethesda, MD 20892
Phone: 800–4–CANCER
Web site: *www.nci.nih.gov*
The Cancer Information Service and CancerNet provide access to National Cancer Institute information sites as well as clinical trials and other cancer-related news.

National Center for Complementary and Alternative Medicine (NCCAM)
6120 Executive Boulevard, EPS Suite 450
Rockville, MD 20892–9904
Phone: 301–402–4741
Web site: *www.nccam.nih.gov*
Sponsored by the National Institutes of Health to provide access to information regarding alternative or complementary approaches to treatments.

Social Security Administration (SSA)
Office of Public Inquiries
Social Security Administration
6401 Security Boulevard, Room 4-C-5 Annex
Baltimore, MD 21235-6401
Phone: 800-772-1213 / 800-325-0778 (TTY)
Web site: *www.ssa.gov*
Provides extensive information on Social Security Benefits
including Social Security Disability (SSD), Medicare, Supple-
mental Security Income (SSI), contact information for state
Medicaid offices, and much more. You may be able to apply
online to these programs, and even check your claim status.

U.S. Department of Health and Human Services (HHS)
200 Independence Avenue
Washington, D.C. 20201
Web site: *www.hhs.gov*
HHS provides information on many topics, including Medicare,
Medicaid, childcare and health initiatives, referrals to informa-
tion on cancer, and much more.

Online Resources

American Academy of Dermatology: Skin Cancer News
www.aad.org/SkinCancerNews/WhatIsSkinCancer
Site provided by the American Academy of Dermatology with
general information about skin cancer.

CancerEducation.com
www.cancereducation.com
Provides information through MedClips streaming audio/video
presentations.

CancerLinks
www.CancerLinks.org
This site is simply a list of links specific to various types of cancer.
The site is constantly updated, providing the latest list of links
available. This is a great starting place for beginning an online
search about cancer.

Cancer News on the Net

www.cancernews.com

Provides patients and their families with the latest information on cancer diagnosis and treatment.

CancerSource.com

www.CancerSource.com

The site provides free cancer resources to medical professionals and patients.

Melanoma.com

www.melanoma.com

Site for patients with melanoma who are being treated with Intron A. Provided by the Shering Corporation.

Melanoma Education Foundation

www.skincheck.com

Site dedicated to melanoma prevention.

Melanoma Patient Information Page

www.mpip.org

Provides a research library, clinical trial center, patient registry, bulletin board, and chat room.

National Cancer Institute (NCI) Support Information

www.cancer.gov/cancer_information

Web site with information regarding all forms of cancer including skin cancer.

National Center for Chronic Disease Prevention and Health Promotion

www.cdc.gov/ChooseYourCover

Site with information on how to prevent skin cancer.

Specific Topics

Sunless.com

www.sunless.com

A web resource providing information on tanning products and skin care in general.

Sunprotection.org
www.sunprotection.org
A site maintained by L'Oreal that addresses issues about sun safety and skin protection in a format for children.

Sun Safety Info
www.americansun.org/pages/sunsafetyinfo.htm
An excellent site with lots of information and downloadable guides.

Tanning Taboo
www.kidshealth.org/teen/safety/safebasics.tanning.html
A site that addresses the tanning issue for teens.

Clinical Trials Information

CancerNet Clinical Trials Listings
Web site: *www.cancernet.nci.nih.gov/trialsrch.shtml*
National Cancer Institute search engine for clinical trials listed in the NCI PDQ listing

NCI Clinical Trials and Insurance Coverage
Web site: *cancertrials.nci.nih.gov/understanding/indepth/insurance/index.html*
Excellent in-depth guide to clinical trials insurance issues.

Skin Cancer Resources Directory
Web site: *www.cancerindex.org/clinks2s.htm*
Provides links to many sites related to melanoma and non-melanoma skin cancer.

Publications

Finn R. *Cancer Clinical Trials: Experimental Treatments & How They Can Help You.* O'Reilly & Associates, 1999.
Mulay M. *Making the Decision: A Cancer Patient's Guide to Clinical Trials.* Jones and Bartlett Publishers, 2002.

Coping With Cancer
Pamphlets
American Cancer Society. (800–ACS–2345, or order from the "Bookstore" online at *www.cancer.org*.)

"Caring for the Patient with Cancer at Home: A Guide for Patients and Families"

"Our Mom Has Cancer"

"American Cancer Society's Health Eating Cookbook, 2nd Edition"

"Caregiving"

"Cancer in the Family"

National Cancer Institute (*www.nci.nih.gov*; 800–4–CANCER)

"Chemotherapy and You: A Guide to Self-Help During Treatment"

"Eating Hints for Cancer Patients Before, During, and After Treatment"

"Get Relief From Cancer Pain"

"Helping Yourself During Chemotherapy"

"Questions and Answers About Pain Control: A Guide for People with Cancer and Their Families"

"Taking Time: Support for People With Cancer and the People Who Care About Them"

"Taking Part in Clinical Trials: What Cancer Patients Need to Know"

"Radiation Therapy and You: A Guide to Self-Help During Cancer Treatment"

Available in Spanish:

"Datos sobre el tratamiento de quimioterapia contra el cancer"

"El tratamiento de radioterapia; guia para el paciente durante el tratamiento"

"¿En qué consisten los estudios clínicos? Un folleto para los pacientes de cáncer"

National Comprehensive Cancer Network (*www.nccn.org*; 888–909–NCCN)

"Cancer Pain Treatment Guidelines for Patients"

"Nausea and Vomiting Treatment Guidelines for Patient with
  Cancer"
Available in Spanish:
"El dolor asociado con el cáncer"

Support Organizations for Cancer Patients

National Coalition for Cancer Survivorship (NCCS)
1010 Wayne Avenue, 5th Floor
Silver Spring, MD 20910
Phone: 877–NCCS–YES
Web site: *www.canceradvocacy.org*

R.A. Bloch National Cancer Foundation
4400 Main Street
Kansas City, MO 64111
Phone: 816–932–8453 / 800–433–0464
Web site: *www.blochcancer.org*
Provides Bloch-authored cancer books free of charge, a multidis-
  ciplinary referral service, and patient-to-patient phone support.

Vital Options International
15060 Ventura Boulevard, Suite 211
Sherman Oaks, CA 91403
Phone: 818–788–5225
Web site: *www.vitaloptions.org*
Produces "The Group Room," a weekly syndicated radio call-in
  show (with simultaneous webcast) covering important and
  timely topics in cancer.

Wellness Community
35 East Seventh Street, Suite 412
Cincinnati, OH 45202
Phone: 513–421–7111 / 888–793-WELL
Web site: *www.wellness-community.org*
Provides educational programs and support groups for people
  with cancer and their families.

Books

Harpham WS. *After Cancer: A Guide to Your New Life*. W.W. Norton & Company, 1994.

Holland J, Lewis S. *The Human Side of Cancer: Living With Hope, Coping With Uncertainty*. HarperCollins, 2000.

Margolis S., ed. *The Johns Hopkins Consumer Guide to Medical Tests: What You Can Expect, How You Should Prepare, What Your Results Mean*. The Johns Hopkins University Press, 2001.

McCue K. *How to Help Children Through a Parent's Serious Illness*. St. Martin's/Griffin, 1996.

Drugs/Medications

MEDLINEplus: Drug Information

Web site: *www.medlineplus.gov* (Click on the "drug information" button.)

A guide to over 9,000 prescription and over-the-counter medications provided by U.S. Pharmacopeia (USP).

Consumers Guide to Cancer Drugs. American Cancer Society, 2000.

Financial, Legal, and Insurance Information

(see also **Government Agencies** under **Organizations** for contact information for HRSI, SSA, and other agencies that assist cancer patients with financial problems)

Americans with Disabilities Act (U.S. Department of Justice)
Web page: *www.usdoj.gov/crt/ada/adahom1.htm*

Cancer Legal Resource Center
919 S. Albany Street
Los Angeles, CA 90019–10015
Phone: 213–736–1455
A joint program of Loyola Law School and the Western Law Center for Disability Rights. Provides information and educational outreach on cancer-related legal issues to people with cancer and others impacted by the disease.

Centers for Medicare & Medicaid Services (CMS)
(formerly the Health Care Financing Administration [HCFA])
Web site: *cms.hhs.gov*
Oversees administration of:
* **Medicare** – federal health insurance program for people 65 years or older and some disabled people under 65 years.
  Phone: 800–633–4227
  Web site: *www.medicare.gov*
* **Medicaid** – federal-state health insurance program for certain low-income people. Contact your state Medicaid offices for further information.
  Web site: *www.hcfa.gov/medicaid/medicaid.htm*
* **Health Insurance Portability and Accountability Act (HIPAA)** – insurance reform that may lower your chance of losing existing coverage, ease your ability to switch health plans and/or help you buy coverage on your own if you lose your employer's plan and have no other coverage available.
  Web site: *cms.hhs.gov* (Enter "HIPAA" in the search box.)

Family and Medical Leave Act (FMLA)
Web site: *www.dol.gov/dol/esa/fmla.htm*
U.S. Department of Labor web page providing information about the Family and Medical Leave Act (FMLA).

The American Cancer Society (*www.cancer.org*)
Search using keyword "insurance." Provides information to help you understand your coverage and legal protections, in addition to how to find possible financial assistance.

Health Insurance Association of America (HIAA)
1201 F Street, NW, Suite 500
Washington, DC 20003–1204
Phone: 202–824–1600
Web site: *www.hiaa.org*
An organization representing the health insurance industry. Publishes guides for consumers and many health insurance related topics (click on "Consumer Information").

National Coalition for Cancer Survivorship
(*www.canscarch.org*, 1–877–NCCS–YES). "Working It Out:
Your Employment Rights As a Cancer Survivor"
"What Cancer Survivors Need to Know About Health Insurance."

National Hospice and Palliative Care Organization (NHPCO)
1700 Diagonal Road, Suite 625
Alexandria, VA 22314
Phone: 800–658–8898
Web site: *www.nhpco.org*
Provides information on hospice services nationally, including
information on communication about hospice, insurance coverage and locating hospice services.

Patient Advocate Foundation
753 Thimble Shoals Boulevard, Suite B
Newport News, VA 23606
Phone: 800–532–5274
Web site: *www.patientadvocate.org*
Nonprofit organization helps patients to resolve insurance, debt,
and job discrimination matters relative to cancer. Patient
resources include: "The National Financial Resources Guidebook for Patient: A State-by-State Directory," "Your Guide to
the Appeals Process and the Managed Care Answer Guide,"
among others.

Publications

Landay, David. *Be Prepared: The Complete Financial, Legal, and
Practical Guide for Living with a Life-Challenging Condition.* St.
Martin's Press, 2000.

The Department of Health and Human Services of the U.S.
government publishes a pamphlet called "Guide to Health
Insurance for People with Medicare." For more information,
refer to the HHS contact information in the **Government
Agencies** section above. Individual states' HHS departments
may also have publications useful for cancer patients; check
local listings for information on how to contact state Health
and Human Services departments.

Physician Qualifications

The American Board of Medical Specialties
Web site: *www.abms.org*
Click on the "who's certified" button and search by physician
name or by specialty.

AMA Physician Select (American Medical Association):
Web site: *www.ama-assn.org/aps/amahg.htm*
AMA database of demographic and professional information on
individual physicians in the United States.

Translation Services

LanguageLine Services
1 Lower Ragsdale Drive, Building 2
Monterey, CA 93940
Phone: 800–752–0093 ext. 196
Web site: *www.languageline.com*
The "Personal Interpreter" is a "pay-as-you-go service that allows
you to access interpreters in more than 140 languages from any
phone, 24 hours a day, 7 days a week, 365 days a year" (web
site). There is a fee to use these services if your hospital does
not have a contract with the company; you can use a credit card
to pay. The web site also provides a description of the services
provided, including document translation.

Treatment Locators: Physicians and Hospitals

AIM DocFinder (State Medical Board Executive Directors)
Web site: *www.docboard.org*
Nonprofit organization providing a health professional licensing
database.

Best Hospitals Finder (U.S. News & World Report):
Web site: *www.usnews.com/usnews/nycu/health/hosptl/tophosp.htm*
The U.S. News hospital rankings are designed to assist patients
in their search for the highest level of medical care. Database is
searchable by specialty, including the top cancer hospitals
(*www.usnews.com/usnews/nycu/health/hosptl/rankings/
specihqcanc.htm*) or by geographic region.

National Cancer Institute Designated Cancer Centers
Web site: *www.cancer.gov/clinicaltrials/finding/NCI-cancer-
centers/map*
Directory of NCI-designated Cancer Centers, 58 research-ori-
ented U.S. institutions recognized for scientific excellence and
extensive cancer resources. Listings feature phone numbers,
web site links, and a brief summary of web site resources.

Approved Hospital Cancer Program
Commission on Cancer of the American College of Surgeons
Web site: *www.facs.org/public_info/yourhealth/aahcp.html*
The Approvals Program of the Commission on Cancer surveys
hospitals, treatment centers, and other facilities according to
standards set by the Committee on Approvals, which recom-
mends approval awards in specific categories based on these
surveys. A hospital that has received approval has voluntarily
committed itself to providing the best in diagnosis and treatment of cancer. Approved hospitals can be searched by city,
state, and category.

Association of Community Cancer Centers
Web site: *www.accc-cancer.org/members/map.html*
Geographic listing of ACCC members with contact information
and description of cancer program and services as provided by
the member institutions.

Women & Minorities

National Women's Health Information Center
8550 Arlington Boulevard, Suite 300
Fairfax, VA 22031
Phone: 800–994–9662
Web site: *www.4women.gov*

Office of Minority Health
P.O. Box 37337
Washington, DC 20013 –7337
Phone: 800–444–6472
Web site: *www.omhrc.gov*

Appendix

Glossary

Actinic keratosis: A lesion of the skin that is induced by UV radiation from the sun. It typically appears as a small (2–10 mm) red scaling lesion on a sun exposed area of the body. It is a pre-malignant lesion, i.e., it has the potential to become malignant.

Adenine: One of the four chemicals that make up DNA. Together with thymine, this agent makes up a base pair in the DNA chain.

Adjuvant therapy: Clinical setting in which all visible evidence of cancer has been removed, but the patient remains at high risk for the cancer to return elsewhere in the body. Treatment is administered with the belief that it will be easier and more effective to kill the remaining cancer cells while it's still at the microscopic level than to wait until the tumor returns.

Amelanotic: A melanoma that does not make pigment; typically red or pink in color instead of brown or black.

Arthralgias: An inflammation of one or more joints that causes pain (usually without swelling). The joints may feel stiff, and it's usually painful to bend the affected joint. This is a symptom commonly associated with immunotherapy.

Bacillus Calmette Guérin (BCG): The microorganism that causes a tuberculosis-like disease in cows. This organism undergoes a variety of treatments and is then packaged in vials for use to treat malignancies. This organism can initiate a local immune response at the site of injection, which in some cases will result in local tumor destruction.

Basal cell carcinoma: A malignant tumor that arises in the basal cells of the epidermis. Basal cell carcinoma can be locally invasive, but seldom metastasizes.

Basal cells: Cells found in the lowest layer of the epidermis of the skin that do not make the protein keratin.

Bathing suit nevus: A nevus or mole that covers a large part of the torso. These lesions can be so large as to cover the majority of the body.

Benign: A biologic state of abnormal growth of cells that are not cancer cells, i.e. they have no malignant potential (no potential to spread throughout the body).

Biopsy: The surgical removal and microscopic examination of tissue from the body for the purpose of establishing a precise diagnosis.

Breslow's thickness: A staging system based on the measured thickness of melanoma.

Cancer: The uncontrolled growth of a certain type of cell that has a growth advantage over other neighboring cells. These cells acquire the ability to enter the blood or lymphatic system and travel to other organs of the body where they begin to grow and destroy normal tissue.

Cell: The basic unit of life; the smallest component of the body that can independently reproduce itself. It is composed of a cell membrane that surrounds cytoplasm and a nucleus that contains the genetic information required for daily cellular activity.

Cell membrane: A thin envelope composed of lipids and proteins responsible for maintaining cellular structure. It regulates entry into and out of the cell.

Chromatin: A network of fine strands of DNA that is dispersed within the matrix of the nucleus.

Chromosome: DNA that has been condensed and compacted into a structure that is visible under the microscope.

Clark's level: A staging system that uses the depth of penetration through different skin layers to stage melanoma.

Compound moles: The stage of a mole where the nevus cells are present both in the epidermis and dermis.

Collagen fibers: A thick fiber that acts to provide strength to a tissue.

Congenital mole: A mole present at birth, ranging in size from a few millimeters to bathing suit size.

Connective tissue: A tough, fibrous tissue in the body that acts to support or connect other tissues, such as tendons that attach muscle to bone.

CT (CAT) scan: Computerized axial tomography is a specialized X-ray procedure that takes a series of X-ray pictures at successive levels in the body. They are then reproduced by a computer into pictures that can be evaluated for the presence of tumors.

Cytoplasm: The matrix material in a cell that provides the internal location for many activities required for normal function.

Cytosine: One of the four chemicals that make up DNA. Together with guanine this agent makes up a base pair in the DNA chain.

Dermal mole: Typically the last stage of the natural history of a mole where all of the cells have migrated into the dermis. It usually appears as a dome-shaped, flesh-colored lesion.

Dermis: The layer of the skin that underlies the epidermis. It is composed primarily of a connective tissue protein called collagen and contains blood vessels, nerves, and many of the glands found in the skin.

DNA (deoxyribonucleic acid): A double-stranded chain of chemicals composed of sequences of adenine, cytosine, guanine, and thymine that are found in the nucleus of a cell. The cell is able to read the DNA by determining the sequence of the above chemicals and translating the information.

Dysplastic mole: A mole that has unusual growth characteristics that can be apparent to the naked eye. These moles are typically greater than 6 mm in diameter and asymmetrical with irregular, indistinct borders, and appear in multiple shades of tan or brown.

Eczema: An allergic reaction of the skin that appears as an area of redness, occasionally with small bumps, that frequently itches. The area frequently develops rough and dry skin overlying the reddened area.

Elastin fibers: Fibers that allow a tissue to be flexible yet retain its natural shape.

Enzymes: Under normal circumstances chemical reactions have a specific rate at which they happen. In many cases this rate is too slow to allow for the normal function of an organism. Enzymes are proteins that function in the body to increase the rate at which these chemical reactions occur.

Epidermis: The outer layer of the skin that is composed of squamous and basal cells as well as melanocytes. It forms our first line of protection against harmful elements in our environment.

Eumelanin: The chemical form of melanin that is responsible for brown/black coloration of the skin.

Freckles: Lesions of irregular, light brown pigmentation that are found on the skin. There is no cellular component to these lesions; they are simply areas of increased deposition of melanin pigment.

Gene: A specific sequence of DNA that the cell can read and which results in the production of a protein. Genes are inherited from our parents and are found in dividing cells in the form of chromosomes.

Gland: A collection of cells that produces and releases a substance that is used elsewhere in the body, such as a sweat gland.

Guanine: One of the four chemicals that make up DNA. Together with cytosine this agent makes up a base pair in the DNA chain.

Immunosuppressive agent: A compound or element that can prevent or slow down the reaction of the natural immune system.

Initiation: The initial insult to a gene that leads to a malignant cell or cancer.

Integument: The largest organ of the body composed of the skin and all of its accessory organs, such as hair follicles, nerves, and glands.

Junctional mole: The earliest form of a mole where the cells develop at the junction of the dermis with the epidermis. This mole is usually 2–3 mm in diameter and flat with the surface of the skin

Lesion: An abnormal structure on the skin that is either benign or malignant.

Lymph fluid: Fluid that normally leaks out of the blood and collects in tissue. This fluid is collected in lymphatic vessels, passes through lymph nodes, and ultimately returns to the blood through the thoracic duct.

Lymph node: A small, typically round or oval nodule that is comprised of millions of immune cells called lymphocytes and found in many areas of the body.

Lymphatic vessel: A tube-like structure in the body that carries lymphatic fluid through lymph nodes and back to the blood stream.

Lymphocytes: White blood cells that function in the body's natural defense against viruses, bacteria, and cancer cells.

Malignant cell: A cell that has accumulated abnormalities in its genetic makeup that give it a growth advantage compared with other cells that have originated from a particular organ or structure. This advantage includes uncontrolled growth at the site where the malignant cell originated as well as the ability to leave this site and grow in tissue where this particular cell type is not normally found.

Melanin: A dark brown pigment that is made in small granules called melanosomes, within the melanocyte. Melanin is then transported to cells of the outer skin (keratinocytes), where it is seen as the color of the skin. This chemical is able to absorb UV radiation and dissipate the energy before it damages DNA or other important structures.

Melanocytes: Cells that make a pigment called melanin. These cells can be found in various parts of the body, but are most common in the skin.

Metastasis: The process by which a cancer cell leaves the area where it originated and begins to grow in a new part of the body.

Minimal erythema dose (MED): The amount of time it takes for a given individual to turn light pink during sun exposure.

Mitosis: The name given to the process of cell division that skin cells undergo on a continuous basis.

Mitotic figure: A cell that has condensed DNA in the form of a chromosome that is visible under the microscope.

Mitotic index: A count of the number of mitotic figures that can be found in a square millimeter of the primary pathologic tissue.

Mole: An appendage of the skin that includes a collection of nevus cells and melanocytes. This collection produces an identifiable, pigmented structure that commonly appears as a dome-shaped lesion.

Mucosal surface: The lining surface of any one of the many internal areas of the body such as mouth, esophagus, vagina, or rectum.

Mutation: Any change in the sequence of base pairs in the DNA chain.

Myalgias: An inflammation of the muscles that causes pain or an ache within the muscle.

Nevus, nevi: Another name for a mole.

Nucleic acids: The class of chemicals that make up the base pairs in the DNA chain.

Nucleus: The structure within a cell that contains the DNA. It is usually identifiable under a microscope.

Organ: A collection of cells of various types that perform a particular

function for the body, such as the heart.

Papillary layer: The first layer immediately beneath the dermis. It typically contains collagen as well as accessory organs of the skin such as glandular structures.

Pathologist: A physician with special training in diagnosing disease by examining tissue under the microscope.

PET Scan: A test that uses a small amount of radioactive glucose to identify areas in the body that contain tumor cells. This test doesn't use X-rays.

Phaeomelanin: The chemical form of melanin that is responsible for red/yellow coloration.

Primary site: The site where a cancer begins; where the first cancer cell was formed.

Promotion: A factor that stimulates the growth of malignant cells, providing a stimulus that enhances survival of the malignant cell and stimulates the cell to divide, producing more malignant cells.

Protein: A chain of chemicals composed of amino acids that are linked to one another and participate in many of the body's normal functions.

Psoriasis: A chronic condition of the skin characterized by plaque-like areas of red, inflamed skin that commonly itches. The lesions can appear anywhere on the body but can frequently be found in areas where the skin bends, such as around the elbows.

Regression: An area of fibrotic tissue found in the primary melanoma specimen indicating an immunologic response against the tumor.

Reticular layer: The reticular layer of the skin is located between the papillary layer and the subcutaneous layer. It is composed primarily of reticulin and collagen fibers that provide a supporting function for the skin.

Seborrheic keratosis: A seborrheic keratosis is a benign skin lesion that is common in older individuals. These lesions typically appear as thick, yellow, waxy growths that look as if they have been "stuck" onto the skin. However, in some cases they can be pigmented and therefore mistaken for melanomas.

Sentinel lymph node: The lymph node in a lymph node basin that is the first lymph node encountered by a tumor cell entering that basin.

Sentinel lymph node biopsy: A procedure designed to identify the most likely lymph node to contain metastatic melanoma cells.

Skin graft: A procedure wherein a piece of skin is removed from what is referred to as a donor site and transferred to an area where a surgical procedure has removed enough tissue to prevent it from being closed without a significant defect. The donor site heals but a scar is left behind.

Squamous cell: Cells that are found in the epidermis that are flat and elongated. They are formed from the lower or basal cells of the skin that are shaped like columns and flatten out as they are pushed towards the surface of the skin.

Squamous cell carcinoma: A cancer of the cells in the skin called squamous cells. This is the second most common form of skin cancer in the United States. This cancer is usually curable, however in some patients, especially those with immune deficiencies, it can be lethal.

Sunblock: An agent that, when applied to the skin, provides a physical barrier reflecting UV radiation.

Sunscreen: An agent that, when applied to the skin, provides a chemical barrier, absorbing UV radiation before it can enter deeper layers of the skin.

Thymine: One of the four chemicals that make up DNA. Together with adenine this agent forms a base pair in the DNA.

Tumor: A disordered growth of cells that results in a collection of like cells commonly forming a nodule or lump. A tumor can be benign (non-cancerous) or malignant (cancer).

Tumor infiltrating lymphocytes (TILs): Lymphocytes that invade into melanoma. These lymphocytes may recognize the melanoma and attempt to achieve some form of immunologic control over them.

Tissue: The collection of similar cell types that form together to provide a specific function in the body, such as heart muscle cells.

Ulceration: The loss of the most superficial layer of the epidermis that results in an inflammatory reaction in the skin or tumor.

Ultraviolet (UV) radiation: The portion of the electromagnetic radiation from the sun that is responsible for sun induced damage to the skin.

Index

Notes